Introduction to Complementary and Integrative Therapies for Nurses

Introduction to Complementary and Integrative Therapies for Nurses

Catherine Stiller

Pennsylvania State University

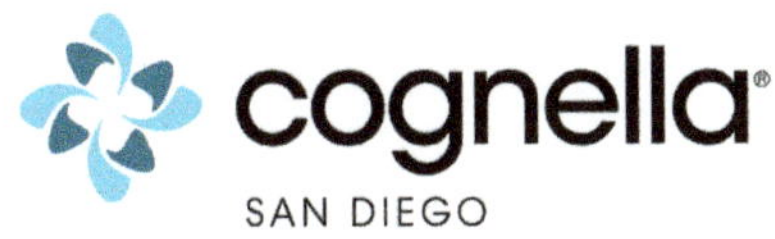

Bassim Hamadeh, CEO and Publisher
Amanda Martin, Executive Publisher
Amy Smith, Associate Editorial Manager
Abbbey Hastings, Senior Production Editor
Emely Villavicencio, Senior Graphic Designer
Kylie Bartolome, Licensing Specialist
Natalie Piccotti, Director of Marketing
Kassie Graves, Senior Vice President, Editorial
Alia Bales, Director, Production and Editorial

Printed in the United States of America.

To my sweet husband Tom, who has been a constant support to me in my quest for new knowledge.

Contents

Preface

While teaching an online 14-week introductory course on complementary and integrative therapies to a group of RN to BSN learners, I searched for a concise introductory book on complementary and integrative therapies, and I couldn't find one. There were some excellent texts, but they were too detailed and lengthy for beginner learners of complementary care. Nurse learners have little time to spare to engage in in-depth reading, especially for those who are practicing nurses working on their BSN, MSN, or doctoral degrees.

I wanted a book that could provide a base for the nurses' knowledge of complementary therapies and a recent edition that was clear and concise and that highlighted the most prominent issues that surround alternative, complementary, and integrative therapy use by people today. I also wanted to see writing from a nursing disciplinary vantage point.

The features in the book include tools that I have found to be helpful as a nurse educator. Included in each chapter are clear objectives for learning, which help to guide the direction of the lesson. Key terms are included to aid in clarity of understanding as the nurse learner begins to explore content that may be new or challenging. Every chapter is structured in the same way for consistency of learning. Each therapy is first concretely defined, and an overview is provided on how the content pertains to the particular therapy or groups of therapies: actions, uses, evidence-based effects, potential adverse effects, the nurse's role in guiding patients in use of the therapy, and types of special education required. The most current evidence-based effects and guidelines are emphasized, and this is important because new evidence is always being discovered in regard to complementary therapies. At the end of the chapter, thought-provoking questions are provided to encourage the learner to reflect on content. This may be helpful to instructors in the classroom and in online discussion boards when the questions can be used to encourage social interaction among students and in turn enhance their learning experience. Also included are optional experiential learning activities because real learning occurs in complementary care when learners sample the therapies or involve themselves more directly with those who are already using complementary therapies. I hope that you enjoy this text and that you begin to understand the immense value that complementary therapies have for managing your clients' wellness.

Reviewers

Jessica Clairmont, MN, RN

Amanda Tracy, EdD(c), MSN, RNC-OB
Concordia College (Moorhead, MN)

Celeste M. Baldwin, PhD, MS, APRN, CNS
Assistant Professor for the Online DNP Program
Regis College
Young School of Nursing
Weston, MA

Kathryn Niemeyer, PhD, MSc, MSN, FNP-BC
Ferris State University, School of Nursing.

Diana L Fleming, PhD, MSN, RN
Kent State University College of Nursing

CHAPTER 1

Toward an Understanding of Alternative, Complementary, and Integrative Therapies

"The six best doctors: sunshine, water, rest, air, exercise, and diet."

—WAYNE FIELDS

Objectives

This chapter will enable the reader to do the following:

1. Define the terms alternative, complementary, and integrative therapies.
2. Describe the history of the development of alternative, complementary, and integrative therapy uses.
3. Describe broad classifications and types of complementary and integrative therapies.
4. Discuss which complementary and integrative therapies people use most.
5. Discuss reasons people pursue the use of complementary and integrative therapies.
6. Describe the potential benefits of complementary and integrative therapy use.
7. Discuss precautions needed with complementary and integrative therapy use.
8. Identify nursing considerations in relation to complementary and integrative therapy use.

Key Terms

Alternative health care: Care that is not grounded in the conventional Western medical system.

Complementary health care: A combination of both conventional Western medical care and non-Western care.

Integrative care: Refers to thoughtfully combining conventional Western medical care with non-Western therapy in a coordinated way with an emphasis on holistic care.

Conventional Western medicine: Care that relies on pharmaceuticals and surgery for patient care and is provided in the United States.

Holistic nursing care: Includes relationship-centered care, the clinician's attention to the interconnection between mind, body, and spirit in their client, and a comprehensive perspective in assessing and planning care.

Thomsonian medicine: A 19th-century American herbalist movement during which botanicals, including herbs, and plants were used to heal the sick.

Homeopathy: A therapy developed in Germany over 200 years ago and that includes treatments made from plants, minerals, and animals.

National Center for Complementary and Integrative Health: Organization that conducts and supports research and provides information about complementary health products and practices to the public; originally was called the Office of Alternative Medicine.

Ayurveda: An ancient Indian medical system based on ancient writings that rely on a natural and holistic therapies to physical and mental health.

Chinese medicine: Traditional Chinese medicine has developed over 1,000 years and involves the use of several psychological and/or physical therapies and herbal treatments.

Alternative, Complementary, and Integrative Therapy Defined

Over one third of all people in the United States use some form of alternative health care (National Institute for Complementary and Integrative Therapies (NCCIH, 2022). They recognize that good health care involves much more than seeing your provider regularly. Broadly speaking, alternative health care is care that is not grounded in the conventional Western medical system, which is a system that relies on pharmaceuticals and surgery for patient care. For example, when one sees a health care provider in the United States, they expect to receive a medical diagnosis followed by an evidence-based pharmaceutical, treatment, or surgery of some type, which is used to manage the problem. The provider may refer the patient to a specialist, who will deliver more specialized traditional medical care. In contrast, alternative therapies include a wide range of therapies that the NCCIH (2022) places in any one of these four categories: nutritional, physical, psychological, and combination therapies.

It is important to discern some terminology that surrounds this nontraditional care. The terms alternative, complementary, and integrative care are at times mistakenly used interchangeably. In fact, there is a clear distinction between them. If a non-Western therapy is used instead of conventional medicine, the term **alternative therapy** is the best descriptor. Conventional Western medicine refers to care that relies on pharmaceuticals and surgery for patient care and is provided in the United States. Alternative health care is care that is not grounded in the conventional Western medical system. **Complementary health care** includes a combination of both conventional Western medical care and non-Western care (NCCIH, 2022). **Integrative care** refers to thoughtfully combining conventional Western medical care with non-Western therapy in a coordinated way, with an emphasis on holistic care. Please see Figure 1.1, Complementary, integrative, and alternative care. The term holistic nursing care is often referred to as whole-person care, and the qualities that define it are relationship-centered care; the clinician's attention to the interconnection between mind, body, and spirit in their client; and a comprehensive perspective in assessing and planning care (Kinchen, 2022). Holistic care is consistently emphasized when discussing complementary and integrative health therapies (CIT). It is important to thoughtfully consider which type of care you are referring to and to use the correct term.

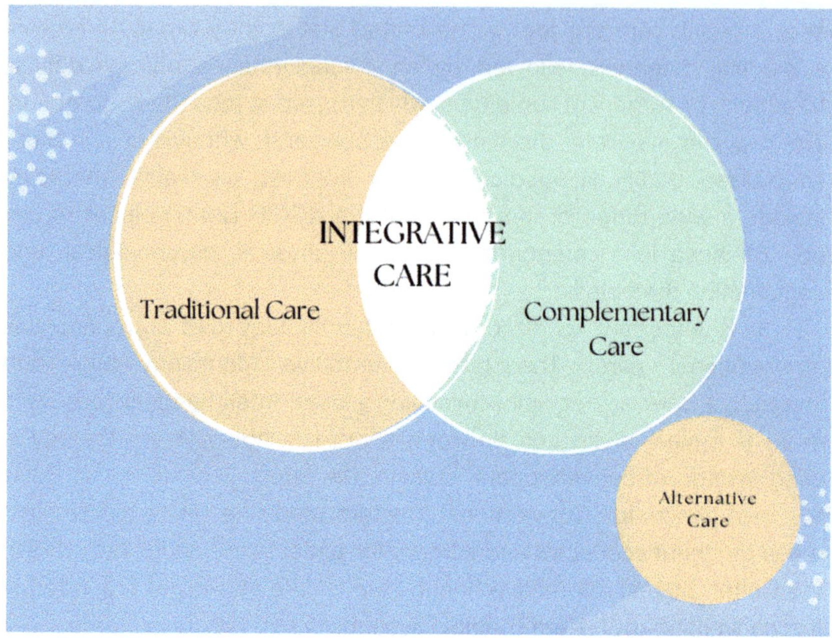

Figure 1.1 Complementary, integrative, and alternative care.

As alternative health care gained respect for use in the United States, the term complementary care was used with increasing frequency. Eventually, as therapies were researched and evolved, nurses and clinicians alike could see the benefits of therapies for clients in specific diagnostic groups experiencing common symptoms. Clinicians began to thoughtfully integrate these therapies with purpose and study their influence on care outcomes. It is important to consider a brief review of the history of the development of complementary and integrative therapies to fully understand the evolution of complementary and integrative care in the United States.

The Evolution of Complementary and Integrative Care in the United States

In exploring the historical development of complementary and integrative therapies (CIT), one must first consider the roots and workings of the traditional Western medical system. As long as civilization has existed, the vital need for care and cure of illness has been present. People treasured good health and looked for help in maintaining it, often using local experts to guide them. In time, the need for good health stimulated epistemological scientific development and breakthroughs. These developments occurred in the areas of anatomy, physiology, microbiology, virology, and medical/surgical interventions (Jonas et al., 2013). Scientific developments have dramatically improved health care in the United States and abroad.

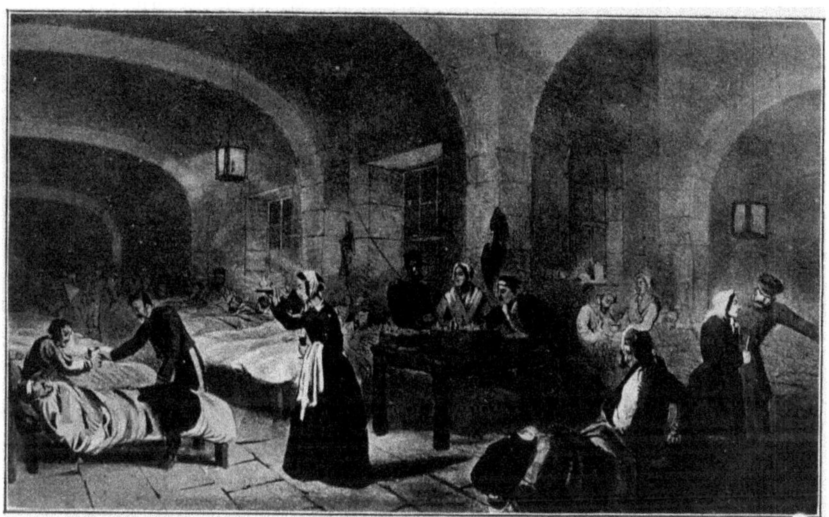

Figure 1.2 The life of Florence Nightingale, 1905.

The nursing discipline was developing scientific practices as well in health and healing, headed up by the mother of nursing, Florence Nightingale, pictured in Figure 1.2 The life of Florence Nightingale, 1905. Florence Nightingale was a reformer of health care, an influencer of the time, as well as one of nursing's first researchers. In her book *Notes on Nursing* (1859) she reported on her research activities and emphasized the importance of maintaining a healthy environment for patients, which included proper ventilation, pure water and diet, proper temperature, and cleanliness (Herbert, 1981). All these elements sound like simple ideas now, but at the time and place this information was groundbreaking.

Along with nursing and science development, health practices that were considered on the fringe or unorthodox were also being developed.

Throughout history, a constant struggle existed between medical care that was considered mainstream and acceptable with those therapies and systems in which effectiveness had not yet been proven scientifically. Professional physician guilds in the 17th century aimed to control the business of disease management. Later in 1916 the Flexner Report declared that only certain types of biomedical science were legitimate acceptable medical practices exclusively (Jonas et al., 2013). This excluded other medical philosophies such as homeopathy and Thomsonian medicine, which were popular at the time but that in turn diminished. Thomsonian medicine was a 19th-century American herbalist movement named after its founder Samuel Thomson (1769–1843) during which botanicals, including herbs and plants, were used to heal the sick (He, 2022). Samuel Hahnemann was the father of homeopathy, which was started in Germany (Logsdon, 2021). Homeopathy was commonly used by persons in the United States at the end of the 19th century (Logsdon, 2021).

Homeopaths carried out thousands of experiments to build up their list of remedies for many different medical issues. According to the NCCIH 2022 homeopathy is based on two theories: *like cures like,* which is a unique precept that a disease can be cured by a medicinal that produces similar symptoms of the disease in those who are healthy, and the *law of minimum dose,* which is the idea that the lower the dose of the medicinal, the greater its effectiveness (para. 1). Chiropractic care and osteopathy were also greatly suppressed during this time, but even so, continue to this day. Although these medical systems were suppressed by the biomedical community, the public continued to use these systems and their treatments, and this went unnoticed by the traditional medical community until much later (Jonas et al., 2013).

In the early 90s two landmark events occurred to the surprise of the Western medical community. The first was a research article published in the prestigious New England Journal of Medicine showing results of a large randomized national survey in the United States in relation to people's use of CAM (Eisenberg et al., 1993). The researchers found that one third of those surveyed were using CIT and paid out of pocket for these therapies (Jonas et al., 2013). Further, researchers found that the number of visits to CIT providers exceeded the number of visits to their primary care providers. These findings were surprising and shocked the medical community. Medical providers became aware that if such a large fraction of the public was in fact using complementary therapies, then primary care providers needed to learn more about them.

This prompted the second major event of that time, the creation of the Office of Alternative Medicine (OAM), which was an offshoot of the respected National Institute of Health. The aim of this office was to conduct research on CIT so that more data could be found related to the actions and uses of these therapies and systems of healing. This OAM was then further elevated in status when it was transformed once again into the National Center for Complementary and Alternative Medicine (NCCAM) in 1995 (Jonas et al., 2013). The opening of NCCAM stimulated even more research on CIT. Much controversy occurred as many primary care providers as well as scientists did not agree with governmental funds being applied to investigating “fraudulent and unscientific practices” (Jonas et al., 2013, para. 5). The growing pains continued.

Researchers and clinicians wrestled with how to best study CIT and over terminology used to describe it since not all therapies were scientific in nature, such as prayer and spiritual practices. They asked, “How does one use scientific processes to study something that is completely unscientific?” The terms complementary and later integrative sprung from many of these discussions. Over time an increased number of researchers with CIT experience and CIT therapists going into research increased. Still, NCCAM continued to be supported by private and public funding, and this further stimulated research and scientific development CIT. In May of 2004, NCCAM and the National Center for Health Statistics reported the finding from the largest study involving a survey of persons’ use of CIT. In 2005 the National Academies’ Institute of Medicine produced a document entitled *Complementary and Alternative Medicine in the United States.* Much work continued in producing scholarly research and documents on NCAM through the early 2000s. Later, in December of 2014, Congress renamed NCCAM to the National Center for Complementary and Integrative Health (NCCIH, 2019). This organization continues to this day to support important research development on CIT and is a great educational and research resource for health care providers and the public at large.

Classifications of CIT

The NCCIH refers to CAM as complementary and integrative health approaches, and in this text we will refer to these as complementary and integrative therapies (CITs) as the term therapy is a common term used in the nursing discipline and includes all treatments or curative processes that restore people to a state of good health and healing. Either of these terms are acceptable, as they are inclusive of both oral products and therapies such as massage, yoga, and others. In the Western medical system, we have multiple types of therapists, including respiratory therapists, physical therapists, psychological therapists, and many others. CIT is also a more accurate term as opposed to CAM, as many therapies did not rise out of the traditional Western medical system and are not ***medicine*** per se. See Table 1.1 National Center for Complementary and Integrative Health Classifications of Therapies. The NCCIH presents a logical way of classifying CIT based on how the therapies are received or taken in by the client. Four categories have been designated, including nutritional, psychological, physical, or combination therapies, which include several therapies that have very different effects occurring all at once. For example, yoga involves a physical and meditative component, so multiple benefits may be realized within the physical and psychological domains of an individual. Nutritional therapies include vitamins, minerals, prebiotics, and a host of other dietary supplements. Physical and/or psychological therapies include yoga, meditation, tai chi, massage therapy, acupuncture, art therapy, dance, spinal manipulation, and mindfulness-based stress reduction, to name a few. There are a variety of therapies that fall under this classification, including a wide range of massage therapy systems and relaxation techniques. Certainly, there are many other therapies or medical systems that do not fit within these categories, including systems of healing like Ayurveda, Chinese medicine, naturopathy, and homeopathy (NCCIH, 2023). A later chapter is devoted to discussing these systems.

There are some more exotic therapies that people know little about and others that are more common and popular. One must consider that the use of some therapies is dependent on the access available to trained or educated therapists in one's region. Use of these CITs also increases with the discussion of CIT in the news media and with providers' recommendations.

It is a great challenge to learn about every CIT in existence and to fully understand the evidence-based effects of each. Clinicians, nurses, and therapists need to know the evidence-based effects of the therapies that they are recommending and at times providing themselves. Clinicians and nurses may use CITs to augment their professional skills.

Table 1.1 National Center for Complementary and Integrative Health Classifications of Therapies

Classifications of Approaches	Examples
Nutritional	Special diets, dietary supplements, herbs, probiotics, and microbial-based therapies
Physical	Acupuncture, massage, spinal manipulation
Psychological	Meditation, hypnosis, music therapies, relaxation therapies
Combination of physical and psychological	Yoga, tai chi, dance therapies, some forms of art therapy, or psychological and nutritional (e.g., mindful eating)

Which Complementary Therapies Are Used Most?

In 2015, a report was published that presented the national estimates of the use of specific CITs, which they referred to as CITs among adults in the United States across three time points: 2002, 2007, and 2012 (Clarke et al., 2015). The study was sponsored by the NCCIH with the aim of providing a national data source on the use of CIT. The researchers used the combined data from surveys of 88,962 adults over 18, in that data was collected during the three time periods to draw conclusions and make comparisons. A National Health Interview Survey (NHIS) was used, and the results were compiled and analyzed for the final report.

For this report, the definition of any complementary therapy included the use of one or more of the following during the past 12 months: acupuncture; Ayurveda; biofeedback; chelation therapy; chiropractic care; energy healing therapy. special diets (including vegetarian and vegan, macrobiotic, Atkins, Pritikin, and Ornish); folk medicine or traditional healers; guided imagery; homeopathic treatment; hypnosis; naturopathy; nonvitamin, nonmineral dietary supplements. massage; meditation; progressive relaxation; qi gong; tai chi; or yoga (Clarke et al., 2015, p. 3).

The researchers found that individual complementary therapies used varied across the three time points, but nonvitamin, nonmineral dietary supplements were the most popular CITS used in all the time periods evaluated. Yoga, tai chi, and qi gong increased across the three time periods, and yoga accounted for 80% of the prevalence, so it was the most used therapy of the three types. Deep breathing exercises were the second most used complementary therapy and were either used independently or apart from other complementary therapies. A small but significant increase in homeopathic treatment, acupuncture, and naturopathy was noted over the three time periods. Chiropractic care or chiropractic/osteopathic manipulation was the fourth most used complementary therapy in all 3 years. Meditation then was among the top five most common complementary therapies used. The researchers found that ayurveda, biofeedback, energy healing therapy, guided imagery, and hypnosis consistently had low prevalence and there was no notable change over the time points.

Reasons People Use Complementary Care

Although traditional Western medicine and the biological model of care and the science that supports it has led to some monumental discoveries such as vaccines, antibiotics, advanced surgical techniques, and many others, it is seen as having a narrow and limited focus by some who have a wider personal definition of health and wellness. The emphasis of the modern health care system is on acute illnesses and their management with treatments, pharmaceuticals, and procedures, and it is not as driven toward the effective management of chronic health issues (Coleman et al., 2009; Wagner et al., 1996).

In recent times there have been shifts in health care that are more focused on wellness, life span considerations, an emphasis on the patient as the decision-maker, and on evidence-based nursing and medicine (Witt et al., 2017). It is no accident that the National Center for Complementary and Alternative Medicine changed its name to the National Center for Complementary and Integrative Health. The NCCIH has evolved in its priorities from disease prevention alone to a focus on the management of symptoms and on promoting optimum health (NCCAM, 2000, 2011). The term integrative health is more expansive and inclusive. Integrative health has been defined as

> a therapy to individual, community, and population health across the lifespan that respects the inter-relationships among all health-related domains including the body, mind, and spirit. It recognizes that health is shaped not only by health care, but by personal behaviors, genetics, and protective and risk factors (e.g., economic status, stress response, working conditions). Integrative health also recognizes these health-impacting factors in-turn are shaped by the physical, social, and economic environments as well as by neighborhood and community conditions, public policy, and social values. (Witt et al., 2017, p. 135)

A broader view of health has been formulated over time with the many discussions over integrative health as used within the nursing/medical community and the public at large. Health care is evolving and includes much more than medical care.

The health care consumer most often uses CIT along with, as opposed to or in place of, traditional Western medicine. There are less than 5% of people who will only use CIT to the exclusion of traditional Western medical care (Nahin et al., 2010).

Researchers have shown that members of the public use CIT to enhance their well-being (Greene et al., 2009; McCaffrey et al., 2007). People also use CIT to manage their chronic uncomfortable signs and symptoms as associated with chronic disease diagnoses, or to counter the side effects of traditional medicine (Lo et al., 2009; Nahin et al., 2012). Users of CIT have reported poorer health status possibly because they have chronic illnesses that have not responded well to traditional care, thereby leading to them pursue CIT for potential relief of their medical problem or symptoms (Astin, 1998).

Consistent with these findings, it has been discovered that neck problems have been associated with the highest use of CIT and subjects with other painful conditions, including arthritis, headaches, and mental health problems such as insomnia, depression, and anxiety, were also high users of CITs (Eisenberg et al., 1993, 1998). Each of these conditions is complex, with psychosocial components such as chronic pain or suffering, and this makes them more difficult to treat. People may pursue CIT to further decrease these problems with their associated symptoms involving human suffering.

One must consider the demographics of those who are using CITS. CITs are used by adults who are mostly younger, more educated, and who have private insurance (Clarke et al., 2015). The typical user of a CIT is a well-educated woman, who is young to middle-aged (Hansen et al., 2014; Harris et al., 2012; Kristoffersen et al., 2014; Steinsbekk et al., 2011). She sees a CIT provider to receive more holistic intervention, and to be actively involved in the care that is received (D'Crus & Wilkinson, 2005; Murray & Shepherd, 1993). She also depends on CIT because she trusts the CIT provider (Beh Natan, Perelman, & Ben-Naftali, 2016), or because she may have a distrust of her traditional health care provider. In a survey of 16,048 women 8.3% reported using CIT. The highest quartile of use was associated with elevated levels of education, Caucasian, and high use of preventative services. The women who used CIT in this group also saw their physicians 7.9 times per year versus those who did not, at 5.4 visits per year in the lowest quartiles. Women in the highest quartile had the most debility, poor mental health, and decreased ability to perform activities of daily life (Druss & Rosenheck, 1999). This also supports the hypothesis that those who have the most difficult diagnoses, which are hard to manage with Western medicine alone, are great pursuers of CIT use.

According to MacArtney and Wahlberg (2014) users of CIT are more interested in understanding the meaning of their sickness than the treatment itself. They describe CIT users as people who strive to know and experience and to make sense of what is going on in their bodies. They aim to recategorize themselves and reformulate traditional concepts of life, sickness, and the body. According to Lobera and Rogero-Garcia (2020), this finding demonstrates that users of CIT aim to be more autonomous in managing their health and this is the "central driver of CAM use" (p. 1279).

What Are the Physical, Psychological, and Spiritual Benefits of Complementary Therapies?

Benefits of CITs vary depending on the type of therapy, the strength of the therapy (one exposure or many weeks of exposure), and which disease or symptoms the therapy is being used for. Recently there has been an upsurge of study of specific CITS for diseases and their management, and this is an incredibly positive development.

The reason this is so promising is that nurses, physicians, and therapists will be able to consult the evidence-based literature to make recommendations to clients for CIT use, to give them accurate information on the therapies that they are pursuing, and to understand which CITs might influence standard treatments and pharmaceuticals' effects. These influences may be positive or negative. Further guidelines will be made available regarding the strength of CIT required to reach the intended effect. For example, some therapies may be given only once, while other CITs might require repeated use for many weeks before realizing the intended effect. Further research will look at the effect of standard treatment alone and with various integrative therapies to see if integration of specific therapies enhances treatment programs. This will be beneficial for members of the public.

Precautions That Should Be Used With Complementary Therapy Use

Just as there are precautions with standard Western medical treatments, there are also precautions to take with each CIT. These precautions vary by CIT and will be reviewed in each chapter under select therapies. It is crucial for clinicians to be aware of which therapies clients are using and what meaning this has for the client diagnosed with particular diseases or going through transitions in life like pregnancy in that both mother and baby could be impacted.

Nursing and Other Health Professionals' Considerations for Complementary and Integrative Health Care

Even though 34% of all adults use CITs as of 2012, it has been reported that physicians do not discuss these therapies with their patients and may dismiss CIT as ineffective and/or unsafe (Clarke et al., 2015: Ortiz et al., 2007). This presents a problem in that many clients will continue to use CITs without notifying their physicians, which could lead to contraindications between traditional medical treatments/ pharmaceuticals and CIT such as herbals and supplements to name one example. Such results were seen in one study of 16,048 women who revealed that only 19.7% using CAM reported this activity to their physicians (Druss & Rosenheck, 1999).

The use of alternative, complementary, and integrative health therapies represent three entirely different strategies for maintaining one's health. There has been a movement throughout history from simply pursuing CITs haphazardly to using the research evidence to thoughtfully choose CITs showing promise for treatment of specific diseases and symptoms. Clinicians, therapists, and researchers have been producing and consulting sophisticated research knowledge on the integration of complementary care with traditional Western medical care in completing integrative health research. Currently there is a wealth of studies being carried out on the integration of these therapies for the management of specific conditions and for persons throughout the life span. We can look forward to the increased creation of evidence-based guidelines on CIT use for different purposes in health and wellness. The NCCIH is an organization that has been dedicated to producing more evidence-based findings to better support the public in their use of CITs and in supporting clinicians, CIT providers, and researchers so they can better advise their clients. Prevention of disease is consistently emphasized, and CITs represent another tool that can be used for this purpose. Many people in the public are using CITs. People have always turned to their primary care providers for knowledge on the best care practices, so both physicians and nurses need to acquire a more sophisticated understanding of CIT use, potential benefits, precautions, associated medical/nursing care, and ethical considerations. That is the content that will be further addressed in this text. Consider using these discussion questions and experiential activities to explore this chapter's content further.

Discussion Questions for Your Consideration

1. What are the reasons people rely so heavily on vitamins, minerals, and supplements more than anything else? Discuss why these might be popular for the prevention and treatment of diseases today. What concerns do you have for the public in relation to the use of these dietary supplements? Be specific.
2. It is important for nurses to know what CITs their clients are using. Why is this statement true? Identify three nursing considerations that you have for your clients who may be using CITs.
3. Describe three ways that we can make clients feel comfortable discussing their CIT use. What benefits do you see in having an open dialogue with clients on CIT use?
4. Are there any real benefits to CIT use? Why or why not?

Experiential Activities

1. Interview a classmate, friend, or family member who is currently using CIT to manage a health problem or reach a state of wellness. Ask them the following:
   a. What CIT are you using? Can you describe a typical experience with this CIT?
   b. Who did you learn about this CIT as an option for managing your health? For example, was it something you read, or did you obtain information from an online site on this CIT? Did you learn about it from a friend or your nurse practitioner?
   c. How effective has the CIT been in managing your health problem or helping with achieving a state of wellness? Have you realized any surprising benefits from using the CIT?
   d. Have you discussed the use of the CIT with your nurse practitioner or physician? Why or why not?

*At the end of your interview reflect on the discussion. What surprised you most? Did you learn anything new?

References

Astin, J. A. (1998). Why patients use alternative medicine: results of a national study. JAMA, 279, 1548–1553.

Ben Natan, M., Perelman, M., & Ben-Naftali, G. (2016). Factors related to the intention of Israelis to use complementary and alternative medicine. Journal of Holistic Nursing, 34, 361–368.

Coleman, K., Austin, B. T., Brach, C., & Wagner, E. H. (2009). Evidence on the chronic care model in the new millennium. Health Affairs, 28, 75–85. https://doi.org/10.1377/hlthaff.28.1.75

Clarke, T. C., Black, L. I., Stussman, B. J., Barnes, P. M., & Nahin, R. L. (2015). Trends in the use of complementary health therapies among adults: United States, 2002-2012. National Health Statistics Report, (79), 1–16.

D'Crus, A., & Wilkinson, J. M. (2005). Reasons for choosing and complying with complementary health care: An in-house study on a South Australian clinic. Journal of Alternative and Complementary Medicine, 11(6), 1107–1112. https://doi.org/10.1089/acm.2005.11.1107

Druss, B. G., & Rosenheck, R. A. (1999). Association between use of unconventional therapies and conventional medical services. JAMA, 282, 651–656.

Eisenberg, D. M., Davis, R. B., Ettner, S. L., Appel, S., Wilkey, S., Van Rompay, M., & Kessler, R. C. (1998). Trends in alternative medicine use in the United States, 1990-1997: Results of a follow-up national survey. JAMA, 280(18), 1569–1575. https://doi.org/10.1001/jama.280.18.1569

Eisenberg, D. M., Kessler, R. C., Foster, C., Norlock, F. E., Calkins, D. R., & Delbanco, T. L. (1993). Unconventional medicine in the United States. Prevalence, costs, and patterns of use. New England Journal of Medicine, 328, 246–252.

Greene, A. M., Walsh, E. G., Sirois, F. M., & McCaffrey, A. (2009). Perceived benefits of complementary and alternative medicine: A whole systems research perspective. The Open Complementary Medical Journal, 1, 35-45.

Hansen, A. H., Kristoffersen, A. E., Lian, O. S., & Halvorsen, P. A. (2014). Continuity of GP care is associated with lower use of complementary and alternative medical providers: A population-based cross-sectional survey. BMC Health Services Research, 14, 629. https://doi.org/10.1186/s12913-014-0629-7

Harris, P. E., Cooper, K. L., Relton, C., & Thomas, K. J. (2012). Prevalence of complementary and alternative medicine (CAM) uses by the general population: A systematic review and update. International Journal of Clinical Practice, 66, 924–939. https://doi.org/10.1111/j.1742-1241.2012.02945.x

He, A. (2022). Thomsonian medicine: Herbalism, home remedies, and popular distrust of professional medical training in 19th-Century United States. Washington School of Medicine in St. Louis, Bernard Becker Medical Library. https://becker.wustl.edu/news/thomsonian-medicine-herbalism-home-remedies-and-popular-distrust-of-professional-medical-training-in-19th-century-america/

Herbert, R. G. (1981). Florence Nightingale: Saint, reformer, or rebel? Robert E. Krieger.

Jonas, W. B., Eisenberg, D., Hufford, D., & Crawford, C. (2013). The evolution of complementary and alternative medicine (CAM) in the USA over the last 20 years. Research in Complementary and Classical Natural Medicine, 20(1), 65–72. https://doi.org/10.1159/000348284

Kinchen, E. (2022). Holistic nurse practitioner care including promotion of shared decision-

making. Journal of Holistic Nursing, 40(4), 326–335. https://doi.org/10.1177/08980101211062704
Kristoffersen, A. E., Stub, T., Salamonsen, A., Musial, F., & Hamberg, K. (2014). Gender differences in prevalence and associations for use of CAM in a large population study. BMC Complementary & Alternative Medicine, 14, 463. https://doi.org/10.1186/1472-6882-14-463
Lo, C. B., Desmond, R. A., & Meleth, S. (2009). Inclusion of complementary and alternative medicine in us state comprehensive cancer control plans: baseline data. Journal of Cancer Education, 24, 249–253. https://doi.org/10.1080/08858190902972897
Lobera, J., & Rogero-Garcia, J. (2021). Scientific appearance and homeopathy determinants of trust in complementary and alternative medicine. Health Communication, 36, 1278–1285. https://doi.org/10.1080/10410236.2020.1750764
Logsdon, S. (2021). The rise and fall of homeopathic medicine in the US, and its continued popularity today. Washington School of Medicine in St. Louis, Bernard Becker Medical Library. https://becker.wustl.edu/news/the-rise-and-fall-of-homeopathic-medicine-in-the-us-and-its-continued-popularity-today/
MacArtney, J. I., & Wahlberg, A. (2014). The problem of complementary and alternative medicine use today: Eyes half closed? Qualitative Health Research, 24(1), 114–123. https://doi.org/10.1177/1049732313518977
McCaffrey, A. M., Pugh, G. F., & O'Connor, B. B. (2007). Understanding patient preference for integrative medical care: results from patient focus groups. Journal of General Internal Medicine, 22(11), 1500–1505. https://doi.org/10.1007/s11606-007-0302-5
Murray, J., & Shepherd, S. (1993). Alternative or additional medicine? An exploratory study in general practice. Social Science & Medicine, 37(8), 983–988. https://doi.org/10.1016/0277-9536(93)90432-4
Nahin, R. L., Dahlhamer, J. M., & Stussman, B. J. (2010). Health need and the use of alternative medicine among adults who do not use conventional medicine. BMC Health Services Research, 10, 220. https://doi.org/10.1186/1472-6963-10-220
National Center for Complementary and Integrative Health. (2022). Homeopathy: What you need to know. https://www.nccih.nih.gov/health/homeopathy
National Center for Complementary and Integrative Health. (2023, June). Be an informed consumer. https://www.nccih.nih.gov/health/be-an-informed-consumer
Nightingale, F. (1859). Notes on nursing: What it is, and what it is not. Lippincott.
Ortiz, B. I., Shields, K. M., Clauson, K. A., & Clay, P. G. (2007). Complementary and alternative medicine use among Hispanics in the United States. Annals of Pharmacotherapy, 41(6), 994–1004. https://doi.org/10.1345/aph.1h600
Steinsbekk, A., Rise, M. B., & Johnsen, R. (2011). Changes among male and female visitors to practitioners of complementary and alternative medicine in a large adult Norwegian population from 1997 to 2008. BMC Complementary and Alternative Medicine, 11, 61 http://www.biomedcentral.com/1472-6882/11/61
Wagner, E. H., Austin, B. T., & Von Korff, M. (1996). Organizing Care for Patients with Chronic Illness. The Milbank Quarterly, 74(4), 511–544. https://doi.org/10.2307/3350391
Witt, C. M., Chiaramonte, D., Berman, S., Chesney, M. A., Kaplan, G. A., Stange, K. C., Woolf, S. H., & Berman, B. M. (2017). Defining health in a comprehensive context: A new definition of integrative health. The American Journal of Preventive Medicine, 52(2). https://doi.org/10.1016/j.amepre.2016.11.029

Credit

Fig. 1.2: Sarah A. Southall Tooley, https://commons.wikimedia.org/wiki/File:The_life_of_Florence_Nightingale_(1905)_(14779827502).jpg, 1905.

CHAPTER 2

Theories and Ideas That Support the Understanding of Complementary and Integrative Therapies

> "By looking at only one place, you miss everything in all the other places! Look everywhere to see everything!"
>
> —MEHMET MURAT ILDAN

Objectives

This chapter will enable the reader to do the following:

1. Describe the traditional biomedical model as it supports the understanding of CIT approaches.
2. Recognize the limits of the traditional biomedical model and current scientific theories in facilitating a complete understanding of CITs.
3. Recognize the overlapping impact of CIT in the multiple domains: body, mind, spirit.
4. Compare and contrast holistic and mechanistic strategies for managing health care.
5. Explore people's understanding of the influence of nature on health and wellness.
6. Relate how holism is central in the understanding CIT actions.
7. Describe how energy-based theories explain specific CIT actions.
8. Describe nursing theories that are used to explain CIT actions.
9. Identify spiritual beliefs that influence the understanding of CITs.
10. Recognize the difference between a care versus cure model of health care.

Key Terms

The biomedical model of care: A theoretical framework that emphasizes the physical aspects of disease and illness. It is a reductionist approach that views disease as a deviation from the norm and seeks to identify the underlying cause of the disease.

Holistic model of care: A patient-centered approach that considers the whole person, including physical, emotional, social, and spiritual aspects of health. This model emphasizes the importance of addressing all aspects of a patient's well-being to promote healing and optimize health outcomes.

American Holistic Nurses Association: A specialty nursing association serving over 5,500 nurses and holistic health care professionals in the United States and internationally.

Mind-body-spirit model of care: A holistic approach that considers the interconnectedness of a person's physical, emotional, mental, and spiritual well-being.

Mechanistic care: A term used to describe an approach to patient care that is focused on the technical aspects of care rather than the holistic needs of the patient.

Care versus cure concept: Care refers to the provision of emotional and physical support to a patient, while cure refers to the treatment of a disease or medical condition.

Natural therapies: Natural substances or processes, such as plant extracts or the manipulation of the body's energy fields used as therapy.

Energy-based theories: Based on the concept of energy, which is believed to be the fundamental force that influences the health and well-being of an individual.

Spirit: The unique spirit of an individual that is their life force and the essence of energy of their being; a force that allows people to transcend the natural laws and order of life, allowing access to a transcendent dimension.

Nursing theory: Includes a group of concepts that can be tested in nursing practice.

Conceptual model: A collection of interrelated concepts that provides direction for nursing practice.

Introduction to Theoretical Support for Complementary Care

In this chapter we will explore the philosophical and theoretical underpinnings that are at the core of CITs. We will review these theories to better understand and explain how therapies can have effects on human beings. Historically, to legitimize CITs' actions, there has been a tendency to examine them through the use of the biomedical/scientific model alone. Although some therapies, such as massage and nutritional therapies, can be explained quite well using the biomedical model, others cannot be adequately explained in this way. Energy therapies, prayer, art therapy, and many other CITs are best explained using theories from other areas of knowledge development, which at times are based in cultures outside the Western world. It is important to appreciate other areas of knowledge development and to have epistemological humility when approaching the exploration of CIT actions and effects. Allowing oneself to be influenced only by one's own culture and popular ideas can be very limiting in terms of knowledge development. Not all CITs can currently be scientifically explained, yet they have a substantial impact on people's health. These positive changes should not be discounted. To do so is at our detriment.

We will review multiple theories that have been used to explain the actions of CITs to give you a broad base of knowledge and understanding as we move forward. Please strive to lean into this learning. Try to be open to seeing things differently so that you can better understand how the various CITs might influence human health. It may even benefit you personally!

The NCCIH has done much to inform the public on CIT use and effects. This is important, but it represents only the beginning of the understanding of the impact of various CITs such as meditation, energy therapies, and prayer, to name a few. To clarify, therapies not grounded in science or explained by biological theories should be appreciated for the impact that they have on health and quality of life even if the state of current science is unable to fully measure how they work. Let us review theories that influence our understanding of CIT actions and uses, starting with the traditional biomedical model.

The Traditional Biomedical Model

The traditional biomedical model is a theoretical framework that emphasizes the physical aspects of disease and illness (Wade & Halligan, 2004). It is a reductionist approach that views disease as a deviation from the norm and seeks to identify the underlying cause of the disease (Wilson, 2023, p. 6). The biomedical model is widely used in modern medicine and is the basis of most medical treatments. Wade and Halligan (2004) stated that biomedical models of illness combine these beliefs: All illness arises from an underlying abnormality in the body, symptoms are associated with these diseases, "health is the absence of disease," mental phenomena are separate and apart from physiological disorders, the patient is a victim and has little responsibility for illness, and the patient is a "passive recipient of care" (p. 1398).

The biomedical model is rooted in the philosophy of positivism, which holds that knowledge is gained through empirical observation and measurement. Disease is seen as a physical phenomenon that can be measured and treated using scientific methods.

The biomedical model is based on the idea that disease is caused by a specific factor, such as a virus or bacteria, and that treatment involves targeting that factor. This approach is often referred to as the biomedical model because it focuses on the biological processes that underlie disease. Historically, the biomedical model has been extraordinarily successful in treating many diseases, such as infectious diseases, cancer, and heart disease. This must be thoroughly appreciated.

The Limits of the Biomedical Model for Understanding Complementary Care

Recently, the biomedical model has been criticized for its narrow focus on physical causes of disease and for ignoring the social and psychological factors that can contribute to illness. A change in thinking related to how we approach patients and treat them is currently in progress. Critics argue that the biomedical model does "not recognize the importance of social, behavioral, economic, and environmental determinants of health" (Witt et al., 2017, p. 134). It is this focus on the exclusion of all others that leads members of the public to become dissatisfied with traditional care (Seidman & Grinsven, 2013). They recognize that some element of care that they need is missing. With that said, most people use both traditional and complementary care and receive the benefits of each.

Let us consider for a moment illnesses, syndromes, or conditions that continue to baffle those of us in health care, and that have not been found to have a known physical cause. These conditions still do create discomfort, disability, suffering, and even death of people. Some examples included the following: fibromyalgia syndrome, failure to thrive syndrome (both in infants and elders), premature death following the death of a partner, unexplained back pain, and neurological symptoms, to name a few. See Table 2.1, Conditions With No Biological Cause.

Members of the public recognize the drawback of the biological model of care in addressing their care concerns most acutely when they are suffering from an illness with no known biological cause. They may be told things like "You are just going to have to live with it"; "This may be anxiety alone causing this"; or "the tests are negative so there is nothing more I can do." It is often these types of situations that prompt individuals to seek out a CIT therapist. Many patients have symptoms that arise from no attributable pathology or disease. This problem has been well documented, and this creates difficulty for the health care bureaucracy that depends on patients having a diagnostic label (Wade & Halligan, 2004). It is the diagnosis that drives insurance funding of health care and medical treatments.

Table 2.1 Conditions With No Known Biological Cause

Fibromyalgia	A chronic pain syndrome characterized by widespread musculoskeletal pain, fatigue, and sleep disturbances.
Chronic Fatigue Syndrome (CFS)	A condition characterized by severe fatigue that lasts for more than 6 months and is not relieved by rest, along with other symptoms such as headaches, muscle pain, and cognitive difficulties.
Irritable Bowel Syndrome (IBS)	A gastrointestinal disorder characterized by abdominal pain and discomfort, along with changes in bowel habits such as diarrhea, constipation, or both.
Multiple Chemical Sensitivity (MCS)	A condition in which a person experiences symptoms such as headache, fatigue, and respiratory problems in response to exposure to low levels of various chemicals.
Non-organic Failure to Thrive in Children	Describes an infant or child who does not gain weight at the expected rate.

Table 2.1 Conditions With No Known Biological Cause

Non-organic Failure to Thrive in Elderly	A condition characterized by progressive functional decline in physical, psychological, and social welfare. It is a common clinical syndrome among the elderly population, which can lead to multiple poor outcomes such as increased morbidity, mortality, and institutionalization.

The Strengths of the Biomedical Model for Understanding Complementary Care

We need to consider the strengths of the biomedical model as well. One of the key strengths of the biomedical model is its emphasis on evidence-based medicine. This approach involves using scientific evidence to guide medical decision-making and has been shown to improve patient outcomes. Evidence-based medicine is based on the principle that medical treatments should be based on the best available evidence rather than on tradition or personal experience. The biomedical model has been remarkably successful in treating people with many different diseases and illnesses while using chemical or mechanical treatments, and this has changed the world (Weiner, 2006). CITs should also be explored and researched for their impact on specific conditions, but one must keep in mind that some of the treatment effects are much harder to measure, particularly in the areas of spiritual expansion, one's quality of life, relief of pain and suffering, and many others using science as it now exists. This will allow those who counsel clients regarding their health challenges to select a CIT that has the most research support for its effectiveness for the client's specific needs.

The biomedical model is also supported by a vast network of medical professionals and institutions, including hospitals, clinics, and research organizations. This infrastructure has enabled the development and implementation of many important medical treatments. Those who are in leadership positions in CIT are amid developing vast networks of qualified CIT therapists in their specialty areas, such as acupuncturists, therapeutic touch practitioners, massage therapists, herbalists, and naturopathic physicians, to name just a few. This will be of significant help to the public in the future. Complementary therapists have developed professional networks in the specific CIT areas as well as guidelines for care using these therapies. These developments may result in the forging of new disciplines in CIT such as herbal science, energy therapy as a discipline, and acupuncture as a discipline. We may have to develop new names for these areas of focused scientific development! Some may say this is absurd, but with further development of each, focused research, and the production of evidence showing the value of each of these areas for variable diagnostic groupings, we will see new areas of scientific development.

Mechanistic Care

Mechanistic care is a term used to describe an approach to patient care that is focused on the technical aspects of care rather than the holistic needs of the patient. Mechanistic care refers to a reductionist approach in medicine, in that the focus is on identifying and treating the specific physiological mechanisms that underlie disease. The mechanistic approach sees people as composed of a collection of moving parts. Philosophers Descartes and Newton asserted that if you examine the parts, you could better understand the person and the disease (Wilson, 2023). This approach has been an important part of modern medicine for many years and has led to significant advances in medical research and treatment. It is no wonder that the focus on use of this system has been used in medical education since the mid-19th century.

One of the main benefits of mechanistic care is that it allows clinicians to identify the specific biological pathways involved in disease, which can help to guide treatment decisions. This can lead to more targeted and effective treatments and can also help to reduce the risk of adverse effects associated with treatments that are not specifically tailored to the patient's needs.

However, some critics have argued that a purely mechanistic approach can be overly reductionist and may fail to consider the complex interplay between biological, psychological, and social factors that can influence health outcomes (Wilson, 2023). This has led to a growing interest in more holistic approaches to medicine, which emphasize the importance of considering the patient as a whole person rather than simply a collection of biological mechanisms. The evidence shows that CIT users want to be active in treatment decisions, are more likely to have active coping styles, and believe that they can control their wellness. They value holistic, natural approaches to wellness and view themselves as spiritual and unconventional). They also believe that lifestyle factors are important in disease development (Bishop et al., 2007). These preferences are consistent with CIT use.

While mechanistic care may be efficient, it can be harmful to both nurses and patients. By prioritizing patient-centered care and building strong relationships with patients, nurses and physicians can provide more comprehensive care and improve patient outcomes.

Mind-Body-Spirit Model of Care: A Discussion of Influences

The mind-body-spirit model of care is a holistic approach that considers the interconnectedness of a person's physical, emotional, mental, and spiritual well-being. This model of care recognizes that the health of an individual is influenced by multiple factors and that an integrated approach to health care can lead to better health outcomes. The mind-body-spirit understanding of care can be used as a basis for the understanding of the effectiveness of CITs. See figure 2.1.

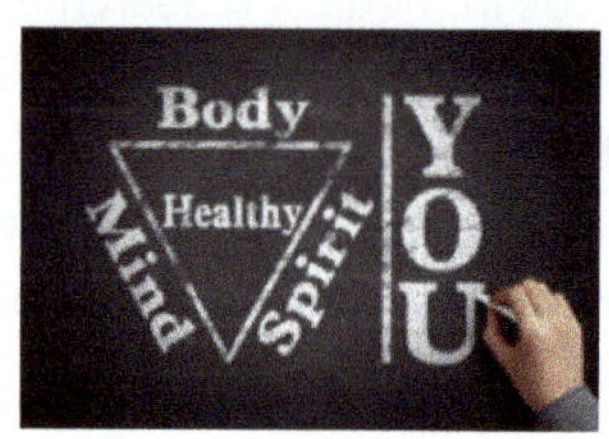

Figure 2.1
Mind-body-spirit model of care.

The mind-body-spirit model of care acknowledges that health is not just the absence of disease but also the presence of physical, emotional, and spiritual well-being. This model of care is based on the belief that the mind and body are interconnected and that a person's thoughts, emotions, and beliefs can affect their physical health. One theory, called the modeling and role-modeling (MRM) theory, asserts that "humans have continuous mind-body-spirit interactions that are both inherent and learned" (Kinney et al., 2003, p. 264). Complementary therapies such as acupuncture, meditation, yoga, and massage can help improve a person's overall well-being by addressing the mind-body-spirit connection.

As health care providers, nurses play a vital role in promoting the mind-body-spirit model of care and the use of complementary therapies. Nurses can educate patients on the benefits of complementary therapies and help them make informed decisions about their health care. Nurses can also work with other health care providers to develop integrated treatment plans that address the whole person rather than just their physical symptoms.

Wellness is a major emphasis in the nursing discipline. In most definitions of wellness these dimensions are addressed: emotional wellness, mental health, physical health, and spiritual health (Hey et al., 2006).

The mind-body-spirit model of care recognizes the interconnectedness of a person's physical, emotional, mental, and spiritual well-being. It is very closely paralleling the holistic model of care. According to Wilson (2023), holistic nursing was once described as a mind-body-spirit environment, but even that description is too restrictive and reductionistic. Wilson asserts that nurses need not be restricted by the medical model in describing what they do, and to many nurses holism is a more accurate description of their practice and discipline.

Holistic Model of Care

The holistic model of care is a patient-centered approach that considers the whole person, including physical, emotional, social, and spiritual aspects of health. This model emphasizes the importance of addressing all aspects of a patient's well-being to promote healing and optimize health outcomes. This approach emphasizes the importance of balance and harmony among these different aspects of an individual's life. Holistic care is a health care approach that aims to treat the whole person rather than just the symptoms of a particular illness or condition.

Holistic nursing is defined as "all Nursing practice that has health the whole person as its goal" (American Holistic Nurses Association, 1998). Integrating the art and science of holistic nursing includes five core values See Table 2.2, Integrating the Art and Science of Holistic Nursing: Core Values.

The AHNA is a specialty nursing association serving over 5,500 nurses and holistic health care professionals in the United States and internationally. Their mission is to "illuminate holism in nursing practice, community, advocacy, research, and education" (AHNA, 2024, para. 1) . Their vision is "that Every Nurse Is a Holistic Nurse" (AHNA, 2024, para.2). Holistic nursing occurs when "there is a request for consultation or when holistic nurses advocate for care that promotes health and prevention of disease, illness, or disability for individuals, communities, or the environment (ANA & AHNA, 2019, p. 42). There are many nursing professionals who incorporate holism in their practice, some who use CITs and others who simply believe that holism governs their way of being a nurse.

Holism has a significant influence on the understanding of complementary health care for nurses. Nurses who adopt a holistic approach to patient care view their patients as unique individuals with complex needs that extend beyond their physical symptoms. This approach promotes the use of complementary and alternative therapies, such as acupuncture, massage therapy, and herbal medicine, to enhance the patient's overall well-being and promote healing.

Holism plays a significant role in shaping the understanding of complementary health care for nurses and other health care professionals. A holistic approach to nursing care promotes the use of complementary and alternative therapies, which can improve patient outcomes and reduce health care costs. Furthermore, practicing holistic nursing care can benefit the nurse by promoting a deeper connection with the patient and reducing burnout and job dissatisfaction. Holism is considered core to the understanding of most complementary care practices.

Table 2.2 Integrating the Art and Science of Holistic Nursing: Core Values

Core Value 1	Holistic philosophy, theories, and ethics
Core Value 2	Holistic nurse self-reflection, self-development, and self-care
Core Value 3	Holistic caring process
Core Value 4	Holistic communication, therapeutic relationship, healing environment, and cultural care

Table 2.2 Integrating the Art and Science of Holistic Nursing: Core Values

Core Value 5	Holistic education and research
Source: American Nurses Association (ANA, 2019, p. 15).	

Overall, the holistic model of care is an important approach for nurses to consider when providing care to patients. By addressing all aspects of a patient's well-being, nurses can help promote healing and optimize health outcomes. Many of the therapies that we will discuss are believed to impact the person holistically, so this model helps to provide a better explanation of the actions and effectiveness of some therapies.

Whole-Person Health

Whole-person care involves care of the whole person and not just body organs and systems. It is now recognized that clinicians need to consider multiple factors that contribute to both health and disease (NCCIH, 2024). According to the NCCIH, whole-person health "means helping and empowering individuals, families, communities, and populations to improve their health in multiple interconnected biological, behavioral, social, and environmental areas" (para. 1) . So, instead of simply treating a specific disease, clinicians should focus on whole-person health and work to restore individuals to health, promote resilience, and prevent disease. See Figure 2.2, Diagram of whole-person health.

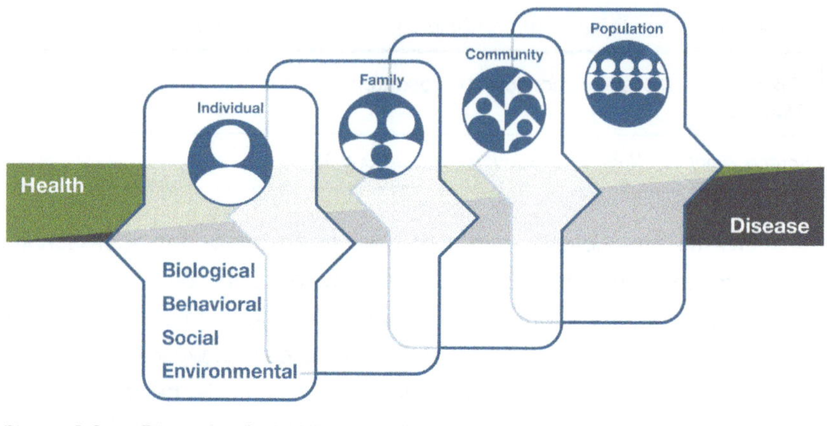

Figure 2.2 Diagram of whole-person health.

Energy-Based Theories and Systems of Medicine in Other Cultures

Energy-based theories of care are an important aspect of complementary care that nurses need to understand to provide holistic care to their patients. These theories are based on the concept of energy, which is believed to be the fundamental force that influences the health and well-being of an individual. According to energy-based theories, the body has a vital energy force that flows through it, and when this energy is disrupted, it leads to illness and disease. Energy-based care aims to restore balance and harmony to the body's energy system, thus promoting healing and well-being. This is one of the most difficult concepts for Western nurses, because energy concepts are not typically taught to people throughout their primary education in the West. The concept of energy is a foreign concept and seems to be incomprehensible because there is no primary learning to build on. This lack of understanding of energy is present in most Americans as well.

One of the energy-based theories of care is the traditional Chinese medicine (TCM) theory. TCM is a holistic system of health care that views the body as a complex system of interrelated elements, in that the flow of energy or qi (pronounced chee) is crucial to maintaining health and well-being. According to TCM, the body has 12 meridians, which are channels through which qi flows. Any disruption to the flow of qi can lead to disease. TCM treatments such as acupuncture, herbal medicine, and tai chi are aimed at restoring the balance and flow of qi. See Figure 2.3, Acupuncture meridians to help illustrate this point.

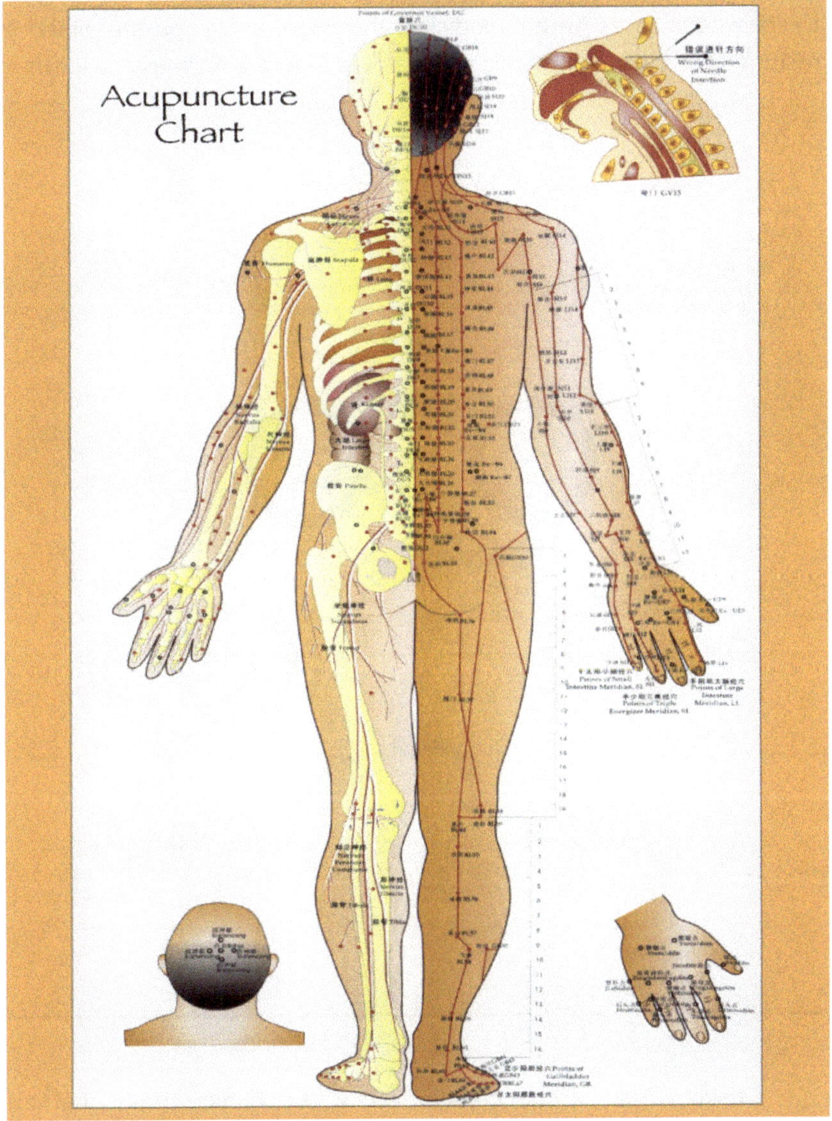

Figure 2.3 Acupuncture meridians.

Another energy-based theory of care is the Ayurvedic theory, which is a traditional system of medicine that originated in India. Ayurveda views the body as a combination of three doshas or energies: Vata, Pitta, and Kapha. Any imbalance in these doshas can lead to disease. Ayurveda treatments such as herbal medicine, massage, and yoga are aimed at restoring the balance of these doshas. See Figure 2.4, Ayurveda views.

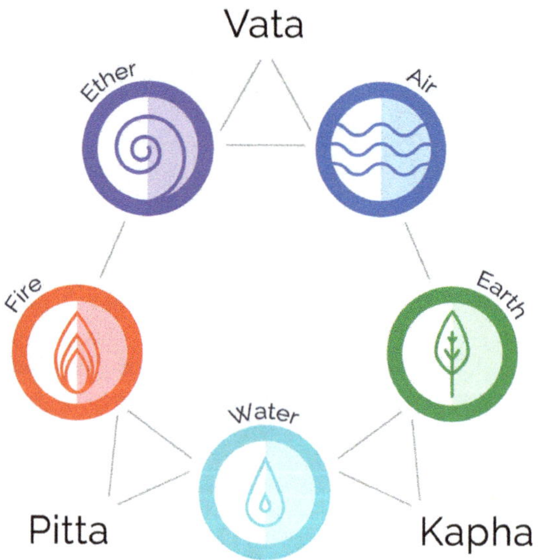

Figure 2.4 Ayurveda views.

Chakras are energy centers within the human body that are believed to be responsible for regulating physical, emotional, and spiritual well-being. According to Hindu and Buddhist traditions, there are seven main chakras that run along the spine, from the base to the crown of the head. Each chakra is associated with a specific color, sound, and element and is believed to govern certain physical and emotional functions of the body. See Figure 2.5, Chakras illustration.

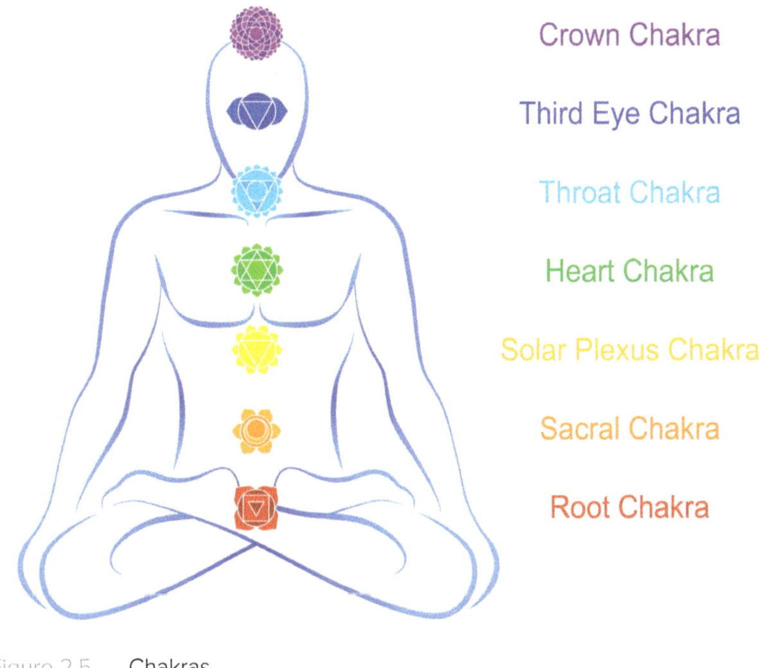

Figure 2.5 Chakras.

The concept of chakras and the energy that flows through them is rooted in ancient Indian and Tibetan philosophy and has been studied and discussed extensively in modern times by scholars and practitioners of spirituality and alternative medicine. While there is no scientific evidence to support the existence of chakras or the concept of energy flow, the practice of yoga and meditation that incorporate chakra-balancing techniques has become increasingly popular in the Western world. Many practitioners of alternative medicine and spirituality continue to explore and utilize these concepts as a means of promoting health and well-being.

Understanding these energy-based theories of care can help nurses provide holistic care to their patients by incorporating complementary therapies into their care plans. For example, a nurse caring for a patient with chronic pain may consider referring the patient for acupuncture or massage therapy to help restore the balance of Qi and alleviate their pain. Similarly, a nurse caring for a patient with anxiety may consider referring the patient for yoga or meditation to help restore balance and calm their mind.

Energy-based theories of care are an important aspect of complementary care that nurses need to understand to provide holistic care to their patients. TCM, Ayurvedic theory, and Tibetan medicine provide examples of energy-based concepts that nurses can incorporate into their care plans. Understanding these theories can help nurses provide individualized care that addresses the physical, emotional, and spiritual needs of their patients.

The Understanding of Nature as Underpinning CITs

The concept of nature has a significant influence on understanding CITs and health care for patients. The belief that nature has healing powers has been prevalent throughout history and has been an integral part of many traditional healing systems. It is the mother of nursing, Florence Nightingale, who stated that the goal of nursing was to put the person in the best condition for nature to act upon them in her famous text, *Notes on Nursing.* She believed in the importance of a healthy environment, including clean water, exposure to clean air and light, basic sanitation, nutritional food, and personal hygiene. Nightingale asserted that all these elements were essential to healing (Riegel et al., 2020). The use of natural remedies and therapies is becoming increasingly popular in complementary and alternative medicine (CAM) and is often used in conjunction with conventional medical treatments.

Many CITS are based on natural substances or processes, such as plant extracts or the manipulation of the body's energy fields, which are also considered a natural phenomenon. Nurses who practice complementary care must understand the principles of natural healing and the role of natural remedies in patient care. This requires a thorough understanding of the science behind natural therapies, including their mechanisms of action and potential interactions with conventional treatments. Additionally, nurses must be able to assess the safety and efficacy of natural remedies and educate patients on their proper use.

One example of the use of natural remedies in complementary care is the use of herbal medicine. The use of plants for medicinal purposes dates back thousands of years, and many cultures have developed unique herbal remedies based on their local flora. Herbal remedies are often used to treat a variety of conditions, including pain, inflammation, and anxiety. However, the use of herbal remedies can also have significant side effects and interactions with conventional treatments, and nurses must be aware of these risks when advising patients.

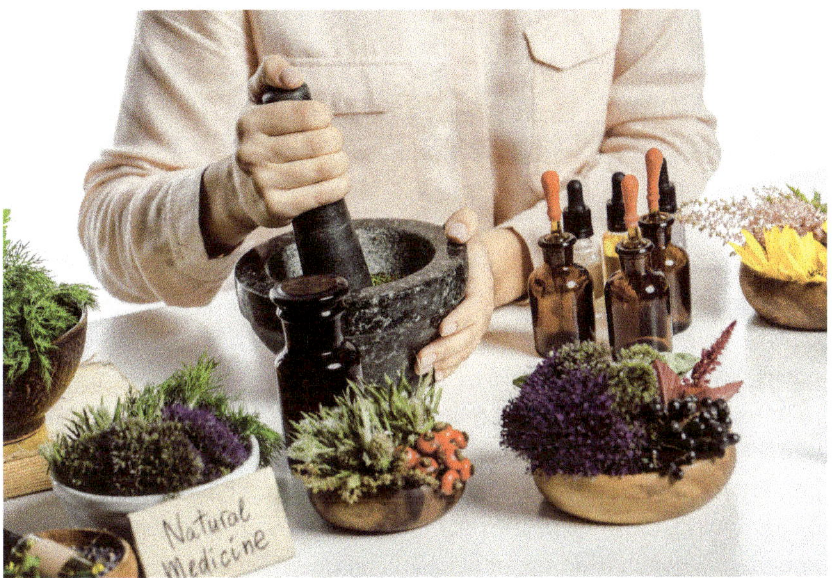

Figure 2.6 Herbs as medicine.

Nature is an essential aspect of human health and well-being, and nurses play a vital role in recognizing and harnessing the power of nature to promote healing and recovery. Several studies have shown that exposure to nature can have a positive impact on various health outcomes, such as reducing stress, anxiety, and depression, improving physical health, and promoting overall well-being (Bratman et al., 2019; Largo-Wight et al., 2019). Interventions such as "forest bathing," when individuals are encouraged to be in nature for its positive effects on health, are recommended.

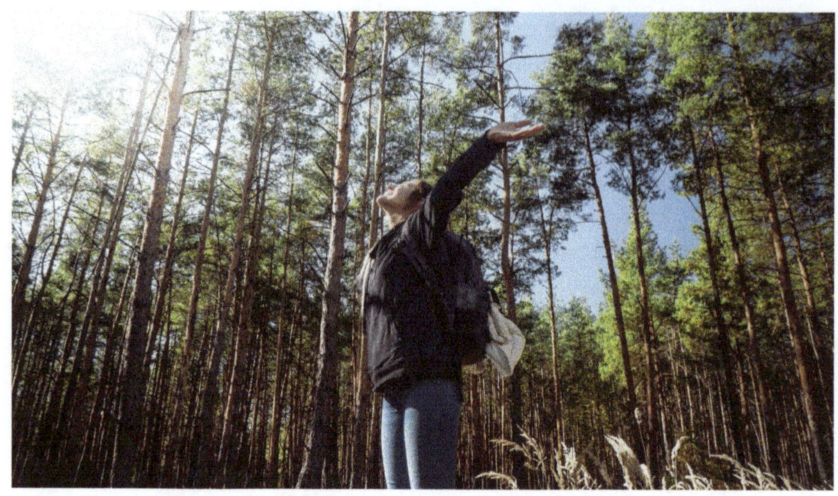

Figure 2.7 Forest bathing for health benefits.

Nurses can utilize the power of nature in various ways to improve patient outcomes. For instance, incorporating natural elements such as plants, water features, and views of nature in health care settings can help reduce stress and anxiety levels among patients and improve their overall mood (Ulrich et al., 2008). Additionally, nurses can encourage patients to spend time outdoors, engage in nature-based activities such as gardening, or participate in ecotherapy programs to promote physical and mental health (Berman et al., 2012; Largo-Wight et al., 2019).

Incorporating nature-based interventions in health care settings is not only beneficial for patients but also for health care providers, including nurses. Nurses who recognize the power of nature can incorporate nature-based interventions in their practice to improve patient outcomes and their own well-being. Incorporating nature-based interventions in health care settings can have a positive impact on various health outcomes, such as reducing stress, anxiety, and depression, improving physical health, and promoting overall well-being.

The element of nature plays a significant role in understanding complementary care and health care for patients for nurses. The use of natural remedies and therapies is becoming increasingly popular in CIT, and nurses must be able to assess the safety and efficacy of these treatments and educate patients on their proper use. Additionally, nurses must understand the potential interactions between natural remedies and conventional treatments and be able to advise patients accordingly. It is important to realize that natural substances can have adverse effects on persons just as pharmaceuticals do. The power of nature is frequently interwoven in our understanding of complementary therapies and integrative health programs.

Nursing Theories Used to Understand Complementary Care

Nursing **theory** includes a group of concepts that can be tested in practice. They are derived from a conceptual model. A **conceptual model** is "a collection of interrelated concepts that provides direction for nursing practice" (, p. 6). There have been many nursing theories that have been developed by nursing scholars in the discipline, and some of these theories help us to understand elements related to CITs. The AHNA and the ANA have identified a number of nursing theorists whose theories support holistic nursing practice: Hildegard Peplau, Martha Rogers, Madeleine Leininger, Margaret Newman, Helen Erickson, Rosemarie Rizzo Parse, Josephine Paterson, Loretta Zderad, Jean Watson, Barbara Dossey, and Anne Boykin, and many others who are moving the concepts of holism, healing, and caring conceptualization forward (ANA & AHNA, 2019). An in-depth discussion of these theories is beyond the scope of this text but let us discuss a few nursing theories in brief that help to support our understanding of CITs.

Theory of Human Caring by Jean Watson

One nursing theory that has been used to explain complementary care is the theory of human caring by Jean Watson. According to this theory, complementary care involves a holistic approach to caring for patients, which includes the physical, emotional, and spiritual aspects of their well-being. Watson emphasizes the importance of forming a therapeutic relationship with the patient and creating a healing environment that promotes comfort and safety She discusses the "transpersonal caring relationship," which is a special kind of human care relationship, a union with another individual while showing a high regard for the whole person (Watson, 2019, p. 63). Watson's theory is congruent with holism while emphasizing concepts that build on holism, including transpersonal caring and transpersonal relationships, harmony/disharmony, and others (Watson, 2019). This is in direct line with the objectives of complementary care and holistic nursing.

Theory of Comfort by Katharine Kolcaba

Another nursing theory that has been used to explain complementary care is a middle-range theory developed in the 1990s, the theory of comfort by Katharine Kolcaba. Nurses promote comfort for the patient through various means, including physical, social, and environmental comfort Ali, 2022. Kolcaba emphasizes the importance of individualizing care to meet the unique needs of each patient. Comfort is viewed as an antidote to the stressors that impact persons, and when comfort is enhanced, people are strengthened. Nurses are driven to provide comfort to their patients in the form of pain relief, emotional support, repositioning, and ambulation, and in using CITs like massage therapy, aromatherapy, music therapy, therapeutic touch, and many others. Patient comfort exists in three forms: relief, ease, and transcendence. These comforts can occur in four contexts: physical, psychospiritual, environmental, and sociocultural (Ali, 2022). As a patient's comfort needs change, the nurse's interventions change as well. Kolcaba's theory directly supports the use of CITs to support all people's comfort.

Middle-Range Theory of Pain by Marion Good and Shirley Moore

Marion Good and Shirley Moore's middle-range theory of pain provides a useful framework for understanding how complementary care can be used to manage acute pain in patients. According to the theory, pain is a subjective experience that is influenced by biological, psychological, and social factors. Good's (1998) theory emphasizes the importance of addressing all these factors to effectively manage pain. The propositions of the theory stress multimodal interventions, attentive pain management, and patient participation, which all contribute to a balance between analgesia and side effects (Good, 1998).

Complementary care can be an effective way to address the biological, psychological, and social factors that contribute to pain. For example, acupuncture, massage therapy, and chiropractic care can help to reduce physical pain and improve physical function. Mindfulness-based therapies, such as meditation and yoga, can help to reduce psychological distress and improve quality of life. Social support, such as through patient support groups, can help to reduce social isolation and improve patient outcomes.

This theory also emphasizes the importance of patient-centered care, a key principle of complementary care. Patient-centered care involves working collaboratively with the patient to develop a treatment plan that is tailored to their individual needs and preferences. Complementary care practitioners often take a holistic approach to care, which involves considering the patient's physical, emotional, and spiritual well-being.

Overall, Good and Moore's middle-range theory of pain provides a useful framework for understanding how complementary care can be used to assist in managing patient pain. By addressing the biological, psychological, and social factors that contribute to pain, complementary care can help to improve patient outcomes and quality of life.

Theory of Integral Nursing by Barbara Dossey

Barbara Dossey's theory of integral nursing focuses on complementary care as an essential component of nursing practice. According to this theory, complementary care involves the use of both conventional and alternative therapies to address the physical, emotional, spiritual, and social needs of the patient. The theory emphasizes the importance of an integrative approach to care that considers the whole person and their individual needs.

The theory is grounded in several key principles, including the importance of self-care for nurses, the value of intuition in nursing practice, and the role of consciousness in healing. The theory also emphasizes the importance of collaboration and communication between conventional and alternative health care practitioners to provide the best possible care for patients. Dossey (2008) describes her theory as such:

> A Theory of Integral Nursing is a grand theory that presents the science and art of nursing. It includes an integral process, integral worldview, and integral

> dialogues that is Praxis—theory in action.[1,2]* An integral process is defined as a comprehensive way to organize multiple phenomena of human experience and reality from 4 perspectives: (1) the individual interior (personal, intentional); (2) individual exterior (physiologic, behavioral); (3) collective interior (shared, cultural); and (4) collective exterior (systems, structures). Holistic nursing practice is included (embraced) and transcended (goes beyond) in this integral process.[1,2] An integral worldview examines values, beliefs, assumptions, meaning, purpose, and judgments related to how individuals perceive reality and relationships from the above 4 perspectives. Integral dialogues are transformative and visionary exploration of ideas and possibilities across disciplines where these four perspectives are considered as equally important to all exchanges, endeavors, and outcomes. With an increased integral awareness and an integral worldview, nurses have new possibilities and ways to strengthen our capacities for integral dialogues with each other and other disciplines. (p. 53, internal citations omitted)

Overall, Dossey's theory of integral nursing provides a framework for understanding the importance of complementary care in nursing practice. By considering the whole person and their individual needs, nurses can provide more comprehensive and effective care for their patients.

These nursing theorists have helped to explain how complementary therapies contribute to holistic wellness in clients and how this can happen, either through addressing pain, suffering, self-care, and other aspects that can impact the overall level of wellness in clients and quality of their existence. Each has contributed to an understanding of CITs and how they can be used to bring people to a greater level of wellness. Nursing has been focused on holism since its very origin with Florence Nightingale's work on the battlefield during the Crimean War. This has benefited both basic nursing practice and advanced nursing practice in that nurses at the bedside provide complete care, forging transpersonal relationships with their patients, and advanced nurse practitioners provide whole-person complete care while providing medical care to their patients. Many patients have reported great satisfaction with care from nurse practitioners. Patients want to be cared for and cared about.

Spirituality as It Influences Wellness

Spirituality is often considered a vital component of complementary health care. The spiritual aspect of the mind-body-spirit construct has received less attention than the mind-body components alone (Kinney et al., 2003). The concept of spirituality is ambiguous and problematic to empiricists who focus only on that which can be measured objectively. The word spirit originated from the word spiritus, which refers to images of life, breath, wind, and air (McSherry, 2008). The word spirit relates to the "unique spirit of an individual that is their life force, and the essence of energy of their being" (McSherry, 2008. p. 45). It is a force that allows people to transcend the natural laws and order of life, allowing access to a transcendent dimension. Spirit also drives and motivates people to find meaning and purpose in their lives (McSherry, 2008). One definition of spirituality originally presented by Murray and Zentner (1989) is:

> a quality that goes beyond religious affiliation, which strives for inspirations, reverence, awe, meaning, and purpose, even in those who do not believe in any good. The spiritual dimension tries to be in harmony with the universe, and strives for answers about the Infinite, and comes into focus when the person faces emotional stress, physical illness or death. (McSherry, 2008, p. 47).

There are many different forms of complementary health care that incorporate spirituality, including meditation, prayer, and energy healing, to name a few.

Despite the growing interest in spirituality as a component of complementary health care, there is still a need for more research in this area. Overall, spirituality is a vital component of complementary health care that is associated with a range of health benefits. While more research is needed to fully understand the effectiveness of spiritual practices, current evidence suggests that incorporating spirituality into a holistic approach to health care may be beneficial for many individuals.

One thing for certain is that many people can recognize that they have a spiritual element to their existence, and they may or may not be engaged in formal religion. As health care providers we cannot ignore this element as it has been identified as a contributor to health and at times illness. In the nursing discipline and practice there are nursing diagnoses related to spiritual disorders such as *failure to thrive* and *spiritual distress*. Nursing diagnoses are problem statements that require a plan of care, which includes nursing intervention.

The Importance of Care versus Cure: A Divergent Perspective

The concept of care versus cure is an important aspect of complementary care. **Care** refers to the provision of emotional and physical support to a patient, while **cure** refers to the treatment of a disease or medical condition. The goal of care is to improve the quality of life of the patient, whereas the goal of cure is to eliminate the disease or condition. Understanding the difference between care and cure is crucial in determining the appropriate goals and methods of complementary care (De Valck et al., 2001) Bensing (1991) presented a theoretical framework and suggested that cure-oriented attitudes reflected the task-oriented medical part of care, while care-oriented attitudes demonstrate the affective dimension of the doctor–patient interaction. Care-oriented behavior helps in responding to the affective needs of the patient and reduces their anxiety by strengthening their coping (De Valck et al., 2001). Sometimes when there will be no cure, such as in the case of terminal cancer, care becomes the most essential element in improving people's lives. In fact, research shows that patients' subjective impressions of their illness and their coping skills help them to survive (Kinney et al., 2003). We as nurses are in the best position to provide care that truly supports patients holistically, no matter their medical diagnosis. Further evidence is revealing increasingly "that psycho-educational, supportive, expressive, and mind-body intervention programs are effective in reducing distress and improving quality of life for cancer patients" in particular (Kinney et al.,

2003, p. 263). These interventions most often are referred to as holistic mind-body approaches (Kinney et al., 2003.)

The concept of care versus cure is important in understanding the goals of complementary care. Complementary care focuses on providing care that addresses the physical, emotional, and spiritual needs of the patient. The goal is to improve the patient's quality of by reducing symptoms and improving overall well-being. Understanding the difference between care and cure is crucial in determining the appropriate goals and methods of complementary care.

In this chapter varied theoretical positions and constructs were introduced to assist the reader in understanding the mechanisms behind understanding various CIT actions. These theories help to explain that the human person responds in many different ways to care, biologically, spiritually, psychologically, and energetically. In maintaining an open mind and a willingness to explore the evidence related to CITs from different perspectives other than our own, we stand to make new discoveries that can have great health benefits for all people. It is also crucial to both guard against being ethnocentric and appreciate that disease management occurs successfully in many varied cultures with great effectiveness. Human beings stand to learn from each other when keeping an open mind and appreciating a diversity of positions in health and wellness. Patients in turn can benefit from receiving the absolute best care that considers them as holistic beings, not just physical specimens alone.

Discussion Questions for Your Consideration

1. Have you learned about a theory or concept in this chapter that resonated closely with your own personal philosophies of health and healing? If so, which resonates most closely with you? Some examples are mechanistic care, holism, body-mind-spirit, a select nursing theory, energy-based theory, or any other theory/concept discussed in this chapter. Identify three reasons the chosen theory or concept resonates with you. Please do some additional research and use three references for your work.
2. Please give at least two reasons it is important to learn about the theoretical support for complementary therapies.

Experiential Activities

1. It is important to help our patients understand complementary therapies.
   a. Select one complementary therapy that you have learned about in the past or have had some exposure to.
   b. Review the theoretical information from this chapter and select a theory that best explains how this therapy works on the body.
   c. How would you aim to explain this therapy's actions to a patient who might be receiving it? Would you explain the theoretical support for the use of the therapy? Why or why not? If yes, how would your explanation vary from your explanation given to an experienced professional?For example, you might best explain acupuncture using an energy-based model of care. Be sure to be specific and explain how this therapy can produce positive health benefits. In the acupuncture example, a therapist would explain how energy can become congested along rivers of energy that flow through the body along (meridians) and the needles are inserted to open the flow of energy, which in turn has a positive influence on health. Some other examples of therapies that you could explore in this assignment include tai chi, yoga, aromatherapy, herbal therapies, therapeutic massage, music therapy, and art therapy, to name just a few. You may select any therapy that you have interest in.

b. Select a scientific research journal article that outlines the effects of any complementary therapy on people when a theorist or theory is referenced. You might use a database like the Cumulative Index for Nursing and Allied Health (CINAHL) or PUBMED. Please outline the research question used in the study, the type of complementary therapy studied, and the theory that was used to explain how the therapy might help people in their health and healing. Explain how the author connected the theory to the CIT and the study. Write a few paragraphs addressing these questions and include a link to the article.

References

Ali, A. A. (2022). Comparison of two nursing theories: Orem's theory of self-care deficit & Kolcaba's comfort theory. i-Manager's Journal on Nursing, 12(2), 34–40. https://doi.org/10.26634/jnur.12.2.18958

American Nurses Association & American Holistic Nurses Association. (2019). Holistic nursing: Scope of practice. ANA.

Berman, M. G., Jonides, J., & Kaplan, S. (2008). The cognitive benefits of interacting with nature. Psychological Science, 19(12), 1207–1212. http://www.jstor.org/stable/40064866

Bishop, F.L., Yardley, L., & Lewith, G.T. (2007). A systematic review of beliefs involved in the use of complementary and alternative medicine. Journal of health psychology, 12 (6), 851-867. https://doi-org.ezaccess.librarires.psu.edu/10.1177/1359105307082447.

Bratman, G. N., Anderson, C. B., Berman, M. G., Cochran, B., de Vries, S., Flanders, J., Folke, C., Frumkin, H., Gross, J. J., Hartig, T., Kahn, P. H., Jr., Kuo, M., Lawler, J. J., Levin, P. S., Lindahl, T., Meyer-Lindenberg, A., Mitchell, R., Ouyang, Z., Roe, J., Scarlett, L., S . . . & Daily, G. C. (2019). Nature and mental health: An ecosystem service perspective. Science Advances, 5(7), eaax0903. https://doi.org/10.1126/sciadv.aax0903

De Valck, C., Bensing, J., Bruynooghe, R., & Batenburg, V. (2001). Cure-oriented versus care-oriented attitudes in medicine. Patient Education & Counseling, 45(2), 119–126.

Dossey, B. M. (2008). Theory of integral nursing. Advances in Nursing Science, 31(1), E52–E73. https://doi.org/10.1097/01.ANS.0000311536.11683.0a

Good, M. (1998). A middle-range theory of acute pain management: Use in research. Nursing Outlook, 46(3), 120–124. https://doi.org/10.1016/S0029-6554(98)90038-0

Hey, W. T., Calderon, K. S., & Carroll, H. (2006). Use of body-mind-spirit dimensions for the development of a wellness behavior and characteristic inventory for college students. Health Promotion Practice, 7(1), 125–133. https://doi.org/10.1177/1524839904268525

Kinney, C. K., Rodgers, D. M., Nash, K. A., & Bray, C. O. (2003). Holistic healing for women with breast cancer through a mind, body, and spirit self-empowerment program. Journal of Holistic Nursing, 21(3), 260–279. https://doi.org/10.1177/0898010103254919

Largo-Wight, E., Chen, W. W., Dodd, V., & Weiler, R. (2011). Healthy workplaces: The effects of nature contact at work on employee stress and health. Public Health Reports, 126(1), 124–130. https://doi.org/10.1177/00333549111260S116

Lee, M. S., Kim, M. K., Choi, S. H., Ryu, H., & Chung, H. T. (2019). Effects of Reiki on pain and anxiety in women with shoulder joint pain: A retrospective case series. Journal of Alternative and Complementary Medicine, 25(7), 710–716.

McSherry, W. (2008). Making sense of spirituality in nursing and health care practice: An interactive approach (2nd ed.). Jessica Kingsley.

Murray, R.B. and Zentner, J.B. (1989) Nursing Concepts for Health Promotion. London: Prentice Hall.

Riegel, F., Crossetti, M. d. G. O., Martini, J. G., & Nes, A. A. G. (2021). Florence nightingale's theory and her contributions to holistic critical thinking in nursing. Revista Brasileira De Enfermagem, 4(2), 1–5. https://doi.org/10.1590/0034-7167-2020-0139

Seidman, M. D., & van Grinsven, G. (2013). *Complementary and integrative treatments: Integrative care centers and hospitals: One center's perspective.* Otolaryngologic Clinics of North America, 46(3), 485–497. https://doi.org/10.1016/j.otc.2013.02.010

Ulrich, R. S. (1984). View through a Window May Influence Recovery from Surgery. Science, 224(4647), 420– 421. http://www.jstor.org/stable/1692984

Wade, D. T., & Halligan, P. W. (2004). Do biomedical models of illness make for good healthcare systems? BMJ, 329(7479), 1398–1401. https://doi.org/10.1136/bmj.329.7479.1398

Watson, J. (1999). Nursing: Human science and human care: A theory of nursing. Jones & Bartlett.
Weiner, B. K. (2006). Difficult medical problems: On explanatory models and a pragmatic alternative. Medical Hypotheses, 68(3), 474–479. https://doi.org/10.1016/j.mehy.2006.09.015
Wills, C. E., & Barrett, E. A. (2017). Holistic nursing care: theories and perspectives. Jones & Bartlett Learning.
Wilson, D. R. (2023, April). Moving to holism: A turn of the cog. AHNA Beginings, 43(2), 6–8.
Witt, C. M., Chiaramonte, D., Berman, S., Chesney, M. A., Kaplan, G. A., Stange, K. C., Woolf, S. H., & Berman, B. M. (2017). Defining health in a comprehensive context: A new definition of integrative. Journal of Preventive Medicine, 53(1), 134–137. https://doi.org/10.1016/j.amepre.2016.11.029

Credits

CHAPTER 3

Nutritional Therapies

"Our food should be our medicine, and our medicine should be our food."

—HIPPOCRATES

Objectives

This chapter will enable the reader to do the following:

1. Identify varied nutritional therapies that are used to promote optimum health and care for common health disorders.
2. Discuss the theoretical rationale for the mode of action of nutritional therapies.
3. Compare and contrast various nutritional therapies, including specialized diets, dietary supplements, vitamins, minerals, herbals, natural products, phytochemicals, prebiotics, and probiotics.
4. Discuss common uses for nutritional therapies in people.
5. Describe evidence-based effects of nutritional therapies.
6. Discuss potential adverse effects to nutritional therapies in people.
7. Describe the role of health care providers in guiding patients regarding their use of nutritional therapies.
8. Discuss the role of health care professionals, types of specialized education required, and guidelines for those who wish to help people with using nutritional therapies.
9. Define nutraceuticals.
10. Define aromatherapy.
11. Define probiotics and prebiotics and discuss their value and uses.

Key Terms

Aromatherapy: "Use of essential oils from plants (flower, herbs, or trees) as a complementary health approach" (NCCIH, 2023, para. 1).

Special diets: Special diets mean the specially prepared food or types of food specific to the medical condition or diagnosis of an individual and in support of an evidence-based treatment regimen (Law Insider, n.d.).

Dietary approaches to stop hypertension (DASH) diet: An eating plan used expressively to reduce blood pressure. People are encouraged to eat fruits, vegetables, and low-fat dairy products while decreasing eating total fat, saturated fat, cholesterol, and sodium (Svetkey et al., 1999).

Dietary supplement: A product intended for ingestion that, among other requirements, contains a dietary ingredient intended to supplement (The Food and Drug Administration, June, 2023).

Nutraceutical: Products intended to have health benefits in addition to their basic nutritional value (Williamson et al., 2020)

Nutrients: The chemical substances obtained through food that are needed by the body for growth, maintenance, and repair (Lutz et al., 2015).

Vegetarian diet: Focused on eating plant-based foods and eliminating animal-based food (Pattar et al., 2023).

Herbs: Small, seed-bearing plants with fleshy (herbaceous) parts, rather than woody, which are useful to humans (All About Herbs, 2011).

Paleo diet: A diet based on what people are believed to have eaten during the Paleolithic Age. This diet includes lean meat, fish, shellfish, fruits, vegetables, vegetable oils, eggs, nuts, seeds, and roots (Lindeberg et al., 2007).

Probiotics: "Microbial food supplements that beneficially affect the host by improving its intestinal microbial balance" and these have been used to adjust the composition of the gut flora" (Gibson & Roberfroid, 1995, p. 1401).

Prebiotics: A "non-digestible food ingredient that beneficially affects the host by selectively stimulating the growth and/or activity of one or a limited number of bacteria in the colon, and thus improves host health" (Gibson & Roberfroid, 1995, p. 1401)

Phytochemicals: Non-nutritive substances found in plants that contribute significantly to the flavor and color of the plants as well as the beverages derived from them (Rudzińska et al., 2023).

South Beach diet: Low carbohydrate diet used to promote weight loss and wellness by avoiding insulin-level spikes and consuming foods that have a low glycemic index (Agatston, 2003).

Minerals: Inorganic substances that become part of the body's composition and contribute to the growth and maintenance of the body's health (Lutz et al., 2015, p. 133).

Vitamins: "Organic substances needed by the body in small amounts for normal metabolism, growth, and maintenance" (Lutz et al., 2015, p. 97).

Introduction to Nutritional Therapies

In this chapter we will address the use of special diets used to maintain health or treat illness. We will also address various nutraceuticals, including vitamins, minerals, herbs, phytochemicals, prebiotics, probiotics, and other natural products that are consumed with the express intention to maximize health or to prevent/treat disease. We could easily devote an entire chapter to herbal therapies, aromatherapies, and any other nutritional therapy, but the goal is to simply get familiar with the wide variety of nutritional therapies in use today.

Those who pursue CIT use are "likely to have active coping strategies and believe that they can control their health" (Bishop et al., 2007, p. 862). They may choose to use their nutrition or nutraceuticals as a tool to avoid diet-related diseases, and they would not be wrong in doing so. Today, it is a well-known fact that both sedentary behavior and an unhealthy diet are major risk factors to the formation of chronic disease. Likewise, good nutrition contributes to the decrease of chronic diseases (Murdaugh et al., 2019). As an example of the impact of nutrition on one's health, obesity has been linked to some of the leading causes of death in the United States, including certain types of cancer, type 2 diabetes, stroke, and heart disease (CDC, 2023). These diseases are among the leading causes of preventable, premature death. Vegetarian diets have been found to have positive impacts on health outcomes such as weight and BMI versus nonvegetarians in some controlled studies (Pattar et al., 2022). Further, vitamins and other supplements have also been found to impact health parameters. As an example, omega-3 fatty acids are associated with a lower risk of developing CV disease and kidney disease (BMJ, 2023; Mozaffarian & Wu, 2023). There is no doubt that in specific cases nutritional factors impact both wellness and the incidence of disease. Many pursue nutritional options to either enhance their wellness or to control/prevent disease. Let us take a moment to consider the impact of the obesity epidemic on health and wellness as this has a direct correlation to the type of diet one consumes.

The global epidemic of obesity is a major problem that keeps on getting worse. According to the CDC (2023) and the National Health and Nutrition Exam Survey from 2021, "From 1999–2000 through 2017–March 2020, US obesity prevalence increased from 30.5% to 41.9%. During the same time, the prevalence of severe obesity increased from 4.7% to 9.2%" (para. 1). A deviation from average body weight readings is indicative of worsening of one's health (Dalili et al., 2020). So, many of the diets that we will talk about in this chapter have their focus on weight loss.

Good nutrition is one of the main contributors to good health and contributes to the reduction of chronic diseases (Murdaugh et al., 2019). Unfortunately, common eating practices and diets in developed countries often include increased fats, additives, and calories, and this contributes to the obesity epidemic. Each year over 5,000 Americans are surveyed and asked to report on what they ate or drank for 2 days. This research is a part of the Health and Human Services National Health and Examination Survey and includes physical examinations (Lutz et al., 2015). Table 3.1 shows the results from 2015 regarding the American diet.

Unhealthy diet contributes to approximately 678,000 deaths each year in the United States, due to nutrition- and obesity-related diseases, such as heart disease, cancer, and type 2 diabetes (Center for Science in Public Interest, 2023). In the last 30 years, obesity rates have doubled in adults, tripled in children, and quadrupled in adolescents (Center for Science in Public Interest, 2023).

Table 3.1 What We Eat in America

1. Less than two ounces of whole grains per day compared with the 1.5 to 5 ounces recommended.
2. Grain-based desserts (cakes, cookies, pies, cobblers, sweet rolls, pastries, and doughnuts) accounted for a greater proportion of daily kilocalories than did any other food group.
3. Average intake of fluid milk in persons 9 years of age or older was about three quarters of a cup compared with the recommended amount of three cups.

Table 3.1 What We Eat in America

4. Snacks provided 32% of all daily kilocalories from solid fats and added sugars for women and 31% for men
Source: Bliss (2012)

Nurses are in a prime position to help people with eating better nutrition and achieving optimum health. Teaching the public about their health is a major professional responsibility, but many scholars are quick to point out that the issue of obesity is complex and teaching alone most often is ineffective. People often have the essential information but still fail to eat nutritious foods in the right amount. Decision-making regarding what to eat involves emotions, feelings, and memories (Jacquier et al., 2012, as cited in Lutz et al., 2015). Many people take on a special diet to gain control of obesity, but others may pursue special diets to manage specific diseases. We will consider this as we review special diets used as complementary for one's wellness.

Now we will introduce a few of some of the most popular specialized diets that have been used in recent times. We will focus on defining each diet, discuss its mechanisms of actions, uses, safety, potential adverse effects/concerns, and nursing considerations. There are countless types of diets both in the developed and underdeveloped world, and it would be impossible to review them all. The focus will be on those diets used in developed countries where the focus is achieving health and wellness or preventing/treating a particular type of disease. The vegetarian diet, Paleo diet, South Beach/Atkins diet, ketogenic diet, and intermittent diets will be discussed.

Vegetarian Diet

A vegetarian diet is focused on eating plant-based foods and eliminating animal-based food. The vegetarian diet contains mostly plant-based foods, including vegetables, fruits, nuts, seeds, legumes, and grains. Pattar et al. (2022) provide a succinct overview of variations to this diet, which include the vegan diet whereby the diet includes an elimination of all animal products of any kind. This diet is adopted either for physical reasons alone or for ethical reasons such as protecting animals or protecting the environment. See figure 3.1, The vegetarian diet.

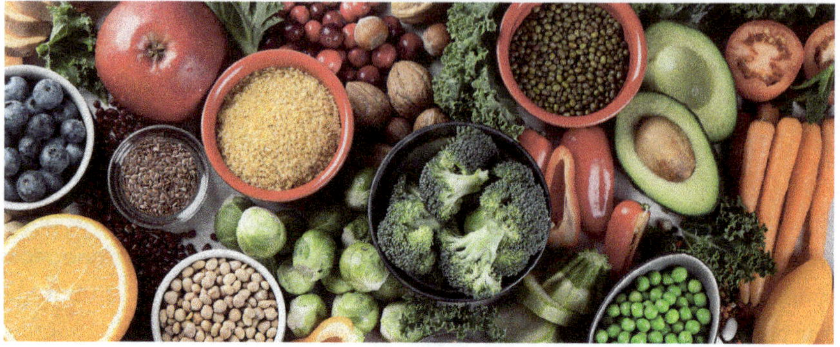

Figure 3.1 The vegetarian diet.

In the lacto-ovo-vegetarian diet animal products, whole milk, and eggs are allowed but meat is avoided. A lacto-vegetarian diet allows dairy products but no meat or eggs. An ovo-vegetarian diet allows eggs but no dairy products or meat of any kind. Finally, the pesco-vegetarian diet does not allow meat or poultry but does allow fish. Of these diets the most common are the lacto-ovo-vegetarian and vegan diets (Huang et al., 2012, 2016).

Another variation to the vegetarian diet is the Mediterranean diet, which is considered a separate and distinct diet but is also plant based and emphasizes the consumption of olive oil, moderate amounts of red wine, and fish (Natural Medicines, 2023). This diet is rich in polyunsaturated fats, including omega-3 fatty acids from nuts, olive oil, and fish. For this reason, it is believed to decrease cardiovascular risk. A pescatarian diet is one that is vegetable based but also includes fish.

Mechanisms of Action

Every 5 years the U.S. Department of Agriculture (USDA) and the U.S. Department of Health and Human services publish dietary guidelines for Americans. These are based on the most up-to-date scientific evidence and medical information (Lutz et al., 2015). The latest educational food guidelines include an educational tool called My Plate, which shows the proportions of five food groups: fruits, vegetables, grains, protein, and dairy. The goal is to help people reduce their risks for diabetes, cardiovascular disease, obesity, cancer, and other chronic diseases by helping them make healthy choices at every meal (Lutz et al., 2015; see www.choosemyplate.gov/SuperTracker. See Figure 3.2, My Plate.

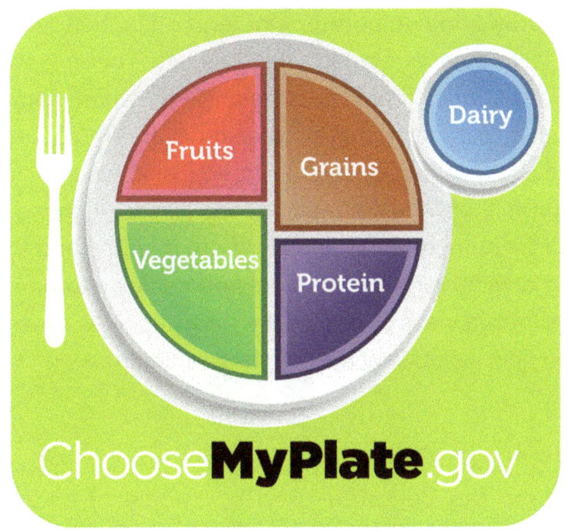

Figure 3.2 My Plate.

The hope is that people will eat more nutritious foods and in the right proportions. Vegetables, fruits, and whole grains represent three sections of the MyPlate tool. There is no section for sugar or grain-based desserts. It is important as we begin our discussion of the vegetarian diet to point out that health benefits occur with vegetarian diets only when the vegetarian eats nutritious foods as opposed to simply avoiding meat, because diets that just avoid meat and contain enormous quantities of foods that are high in sugar and saturated fats are likely to be harmful (Van Horn et al., 2016). Vegetables and fruit are very nutritious.

Vegetarian diets are healthy as the diet helps to promote greater consumption of nutritious fruits, vegetables, whole grains, and legumes (Lee & Park, 2017). This appears to lead to a number of health benefits, as illustrated with the latest research evidence. Consuming a vegetarian diet helps in the maintenance of healthy body weight and blood pressure, kidney health, and cardiovascular health. Daily calorie counts are lower, and the vegetarian diet is higher in fiber, which results in a decrease in weight and BMI. The foods normally eaten are of a lower glycemic index, and vegetarians have greater glycemic control (Viguiliouk et al., 2018). In one study of adults, the lacto-ovo-vegetarian diet had beneficial effects on kidney function, a decrease in creatinine and blood urea nitrogen levels, as well as improvement in glomerular filtration rate (Dinu et al., 2021). The lacto-ovo-vegetarian diet has also been associated with decreased levels of C-reactive protein (CRP) when compared to an omnivorous diet, in a meta-analysis (Menzel et al., 2020). The importance of vegetables in promoting overall health and well-being cannot be overstated. From their vital nutrients to their disease-fighting antioxidants, vegetables offer numerous benefits for both physical and mental health. Incorporating a wide variety of colorful vegetables into one's diet is one of the most effective ways to ensure the body receives essential vitamins, minerals, and fiber necessary for optimal functioning.

Therapeutic Uses of the Vegetarian Diet

Vegetarian diets can be safely used by people of all ages if proper attention is placed to nutrients that may be missing due to the lack of consumption of meat, eggs, and milk products. People may pursue a vegetarian diet with the goal of achieving a greater state of wellness, to reach a lower weight and the associated BMI, to increase gastric motility and digestive health, to decrease cholesterol levels, to decrease blood pressure, or simply to feel some satisfaction that they are not harming animals and the ecosystem.

Safety

A position statement from the Academy of Nutrition and Dietetics indicated that a vegetarian diet is appropriate for adults if all elements of nutrition are given proper attention (Melina et al., 2016). One must ensure that they get adequate amounts of omega-3 fatty acids, vitamin D, calcium, vitamin B12, iron, and zinc (Melina et al., 2016; see Table 3.2. Likewise, a vegetarian diet is appropriate during infancy, childhood, and adolescence (Melina et al., 2016), once again if the stated nutrients are provided. A vegetarian diet has also been shown to be safe during both pregnancy and lactation, with one exception. When specific vegetarian diets were examined, the vegan diet, when vegetables only are eaten, to the exclusion of all animal products, including meat, eggs, milk, and other dairy, has been associated with low birth weight (Tan et al., 2019).

Potential Adverse Effects and Concerns

The vegetarian diet is a safe and nutritious option for people if proper attention is given to taking in the specific nutrients: omega-3 fatty acids, iron, zinc, calcium, vitamin D, and B12. Numerous benefits to a vegetarian diet have been revealed, and it is worth considering pursuing this diet. The problem of low birthweight is a special concern of the strict vegan diet.

Nurse Guidance for Use of the Vegetarian Diet

Heart disease is a leading cause of death in America. It is responsible for killing one in four Americans (CDC, 2023). Elevated cholesterol runs rampant in America, affecting 73 million people (CDC, 2023). More than two thirds of Americans are overweight or obese, which leads to chronic diseases, including coronary heart disease, cancer, and diabetes (Huang et al., 2016). A vegetarian diet can help people lose weight, decrease cholesterol levels and blood pressure, as well as prevent cardiovascular disease. It is worth pursuing as a preventative or treatment option for patients.

Nurses have a responsibility to learn about vegetarian diets and to teach their patients about the benefits and precautions involved with making the change to consuming this type of diet. Nurse leaders can develop plant-based nutrition programs to help their patients in managing a vegetarian diet (Evans et al., 2017).

This diet should complement rather than replace other measures patients use to manage their health. For example, if the health concern is blood pressure, a patient should continue measures to manage it, such as taking their antihypertensive agents and lowering their sodium. If they are on anticholesterol agents, these should be continued but reevaluated after a vegetarian diet has been in use and has had some time to take effect. Patients and clients should be cautioned that a vegetarian diet will not lead to immediate dramatic change in indices like cholesterol and blood pressure but that these changes may come in time. A vegetarian diet must be used for 3 months before it has a modest reduction in body weight (Natural Medicines, 2022)

Nurses need to be advocates for their patients who are interested in pursuing a vegetarian diet as this represents a positive change for them. They also need to caution patients to get nutrients that supply omega-3 fatty acids, vitamin D, calcium, vitamin B12, iron, and zinc. See Table 3.2, Vegetarian Sources of Key Nutrients. Patients who are at risk for developing diabetes should be presented with some research that shows a vegetarian diet may be beneficial for preventing diabetes (Natural Medicines, 2022).

Nurses need to be aware that their vegetarian patients may have more difficulty absorbing plant-derived iron (nonheme iron), may have reduced absorption of zinc requiring 50% more zinc in the diet to meet nutritional requirements, and may have inadequate calcium intake leading to decreased bone density (Van Horn et al., 2016). These patients may need supplementation to avoid these issues. Nurses should educate themselves on what foods contain these nutrients so that they can be in a better position to educate their clients.

Table 3.2 Vegetarian Sources of Key Nutrients

Nutrient	Sources
Omega-3 fatty acid	Flaxseeds, chia seeds, and walnuts
Vitamin D	Sunlight, fortified dairy foods like milk and yogurt, eggs, certain mushrooms
Calcium	Milk, cheese, yogurt, plant milk, tofu, calcium-fortified orange juice, leafy green vegetables like kale and broccoli
B12	Eggs, dairy products, fortified foods like breakfast cereals, plant-based milk, and nutritional yeast
Iron	Legumes, tofu, whole grains, nuts, seeds, and fortified foods
Zinc	Legumes, whole grains, nuts, seeds, fortified cereals

Nurses need to be aware of how to monitor their patients for lowered levels of these nutrients, and they should teach their patients what symptoms to look for. For example, low iron levels can lead to iron deficiency anemia. Knowing the associated symptoms of iron deficiency anemia will help their patients to be aware that they may need a visit to their physician or nurse practitioner to get their iron level checked (Table 3.3).

Table 3.3 Clinical Manifestations of Key Nutrient Loss in Vegetarians

Lack of omega-3 fatty acid	Dry skin, dull or brittle hair, dry and brittle nails, difficulty concentrating or memory problems, and joint pain or stiffness
Lack of vitamin D	Frequent infections and illnesses, fatigue or low energy levels, bone and muscle pain, difficulty in wound healing, and depression or mood swings
Lack of calcium	Weak or brittle bones, dental problems such as tooth decay, muscle cramps or spasms, numbness or tingling in the extremities, poor growth, and development in children
Lack of B12	Fatigue or weakness, memory problems or confusion, pale skin, dizziness or lightheadedness, and tingling or numbness in hands and feet
Lack of iron	Fatigue or low energy levels, pale skin or nails, shortness of breath, weakness, and frequent infections or illnesses
Lack of zinc	Decreased sense of taste and smell, delayed wound healing, hair loss or thinning, decreased appetite, and skin problems, such as rashes or acne

Paleo Diet

The paleo diet is a diet based on what people are believed to have eaten during the Paleolithic Age. This diet includes lean meat, fish, shellfish, fruits, vegetables, vegetable oils, eggs, nuts, seeds, and roots. Grains, dairy products, salt, refined fats, and sugar are avoided in this diet (Lindeberg et al., 2007). Alcohol is permitted in some paleo dietary patterns but not in all (Jonsson et al., 2010; Lindeberg et al., 2007).See Figure 3.3, Paleo diet foods.

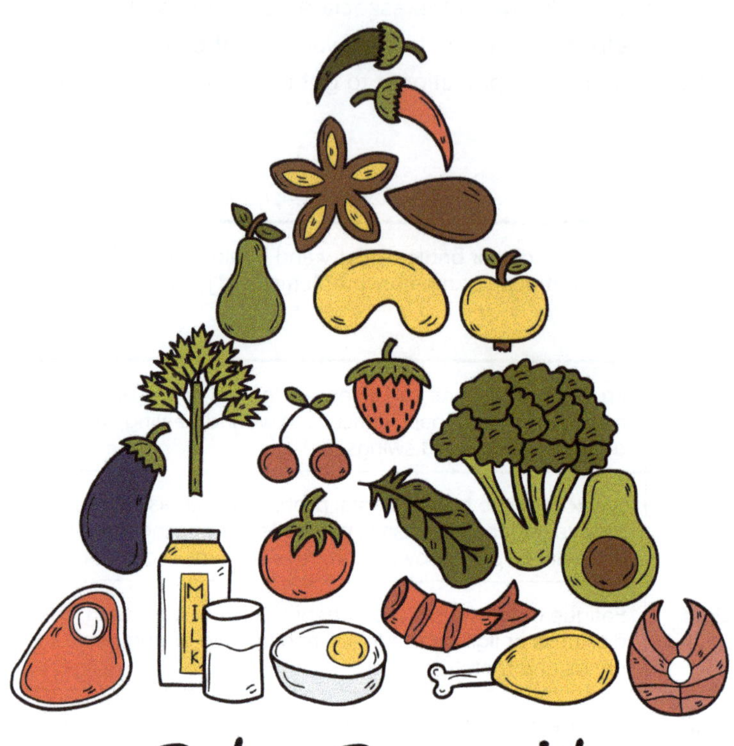

Figure 3.3 Paleo diet foods.

Therapeutic Uses of the Paleo Diet

According to the Natural Medicines, (2021), The Paleo diet has many diverse uses:

> acne, anxiety, asthma, athletic performance, autoimmune diseases, cancer, cardiovascular disease (CVD), chronic fatigue syndrome (CFS), depression, diabetes, dysmenorrhea, fatigue, gingivitis, hypercholesterolemia, hypertension, hyperlipidemia, kidney stones (nephrolithiasis), metabolic syndrome, multiple sclerosis-related fatigue, myopia, obesity,

> osteoarthritis, osteoporosis, rheumatoid arthritis (RA), skin conditions, and skin infections (folliculitis). (para. 2)

Evidence-Based Effects of the Paleo Diet

Proponents of the Paleo diet assert that the modern American diet is at the root of many modern health problems and a shift to a simpler diet as used in the Paleolithic age is healthier. In following this diet people incorporate more fruits, vegetables, and seafood (Jew et al., 2009). According to O'Keefe and Cordain (2004), an alkaline state of the body develops, which may lead to reduced blood pressure, a decreased risk of kidney stones and asthma, and increased muscle strength.

The paleo diet is high in protein, and protein produces the greatest satiety out of all the nutrients. It is believed that this is one reason for weight loss (Jonsson et al., 2013). This diet is also associated with reduced leptin levels and increased levels of glucagon-like peptide that contributes to greater satiety (Jonsson et al., 2013; Otten et al., 2019). Weight loss can occur and then improve blood pressure and lipid levels and lead to an improved glycemic index.

Potential Adverse Effects and Concerns

The paleo diet is a safe diet without reports of adverse effects (Lindeberg et al., 2007). Nutritional needs are met with this diet; however, there needs to be some care taken with receiving enough calcium and vitamin D (Jew et al., 2009). There are no known adverse effects of this diet. Long-term use has not yet been studied.

Nurse Guidance for Use of the Paleo Diet

Persons on this diet have been shown to not receive the recommended daily allowance (RDA) of calcium through diet alone, so supplementation may be necessary (Hoffman, 2017). The nurse can expect to see that those clients following this diet might develop a calcium deficiency or insufficiency (Hoffman, 2017). Over the long-term this could lead to osteoporosis. The nurse should check for signs and symptoms of calcium deficiency and as a member of the health care team encourage their colleague physician or nurse practitioner to check a blood calcium level if there is any suspicion of hypocalcemia.

South Beach Diet

The South Beach diet is a low-carbohydrate diet used to promote weight loss and wellness by avoiding insulin-level spikes and consuming foods that have a low glycemic index. The diet was created by cardiologist Arthur Agatston (2003). There are three phases to the diet, with phase 1 being the strictest lasting only 2 weeks. It is recommended that phase 1 not be continued past a 2-week period because the diet is so limited (Agatston, 2003). During phase 1 the focus is on eating vegetables and low-fat proteins such as chicken, fish, and tofu. In phase 2, a few healthy carbohydrates such as whole-grain breads, sweet potatoes, and fruits are added back into the diet in moderation. It is recommended that individuals stay in phase 2 until they reach their target weight. In phase 3 foods of all types are permitted but only in moderation. Variations to the South Beach diet are in use that involve low carbohydrates and high protein consumption. Low-carbohydrate and high-protein diets are currently immensely popular in America.

Evidence-Based Effects of the South Beach Diet

In this diet high-glycemic foods are eliminated and then later only moderately consumed. The reason for this is that these foods create sugar spikes and excess insulin secretion, leading to obesity, cardiovascular disease, and diabetes (Agatston, 2003). Agatston explains that a side effect of excess weight is insulin resistance. When eliminating "bad carbs" the insulin resistance clears up, and carbohydrates begin to be metabolized correctly. The craving for carbohydrates disappears, and weight loss occurs. Blood chemistry is improved, leading to a decrease in both triglycerides and cholesterol (Agatston, 2003).

There has been much debate over whether the South Beach diet can prevent these outcomes or whether the reduced-calorie diet is a better option (Kirkpatrick et al., 2019; Levitan et al., 2007). Some concern has been addressed regarding the higher intake of fats and low intake of carbohydrates in this diet, but what has been seen is a decrease of low-density lipoprotein and cholesterol levels in nonobese healthy adults on this diet (Kirkpatrick et al., 2019).

Potential Adverse Effects and Concerns

There is not yet enough evidence currently to draw definitive conclusions regarding the safety of the South Beach diet throughout the life span and during pregnancy and lactation. For adults, this diet is safe if dieters are getting appropriate nutrition and not being too restrictive. Phase 1 of this diet, which only lasts 2 weeks, is a time of greatest restriction. Encouraging people to listen to their body first and if they recognize that they are feeling bad to eat some carbohydrates, if necessary, in that moment seems like prudent advice. Since we do not yet know the impact of this diet during pregnancy and lactation it is better to abstain from changing one's diet during these times.

DASH Diet

In the **dietary approaches to stop hypertension (DASH) diet** an eating plan is used to reduce blood pressure. People are encouraged to eat fruits, vegetables, and low-fat dairy products while decreasing eating total fat, saturated fat, cholesterol, and sodium (Svetkey et al., 1999). Further, a breakdown of servings is suggested: seven to eight servings of grains, four to five servings of vegetables, four to five servings of fruits, two or less servings of lean meats, and two to three servings of low-fat dairy products. Snacks are permitted, but only five snacks per week (Svetkey et al., 1999). The diet focuses on lowering sodium intake rather than eliminating it completely (Natural Medicines, 2024).

Therapeutic Uses of the DASH Diet

High blood pressure may result in serious health conditions, including heart disease, stroke, and kidney disease. Hypertension is a risk factor for cardiovascular morbidity and mortality (Fuchs & Welton, 2020). The DASH diet was designed to help control high blood pressure and to prevent the further development of disease. After several successful clinical trials, the DASH diet was promoted across the world as a successful diet to control hypertension (Appel et al., 1997).

The DASH diet has been shown to reduce blood pressure, cardiovascular events, cancer, and obesity and therefore may be used for any and all of these purposes (Jones-Mclean et al., 2015; Mompeo et al.

2020; Salehi-Abargoiei et al., 2013; Saneei et al., 2014; Soltani et al., 2016; Wang et al., 2018). The DASH diet may also be beneficial for reducing the risk of gestational and type 2 diabetes (Li et al. 2020; Liese et al., 2009).

Potential Adverse Effects and Concerns

The DASH diet has been researched and has been found to be safe in several clinical trials (Conlin et al., 2000, 2003; Svetkey et al., 1999). It has also been shown to be safe with children in the short-term (10–12 weeks; Khoshbakht et al., 2021) and in pregnancy and lactation with no changes in infant weight (Jahangir et al., 2022; Li et al., 2020).

Nurse Guidance for Use of the Dash Diet

The nurse's role in managing complementary care diets for patients is crucial in promoting their overall well-being and health. Nurses play a vital role in providing education, support, and monitoring to ensure patients' adherence to these specialized dietary plans.

For patients following a vegetarian diet, nurses play a critical role in ensuring they receive adequate nutrients from plant-based sources. They can assist in devising a well-balanced meal plan that includes a variety of protein-rich foods such as beans, lentils, tofu, tempeh, and nuts. Nurses can also educate patients about the importance of obtaining nutrients like vitamin B12, iron, calcium, and omega-3 fatty acids from appropriate supplementation or fortified foods.

The paleo diet emphasizes consuming unprocessed foods and avoiding grains, legumes, processed sugars, and dairy products. Nurses can provide patients with a comprehensive understanding of the diet's requirements, making sure patients incorporate enough fruits, vegetables, lean meats, and healthy fats into their meals. They can also address any concerns about nutrient deficiencies and suggest suitable alternatives to meet the patients' individual nutritional needs.

The DASH diet focuses on reducing sodium intake while incorporating fruits, vegetables, whole grains, lean proteins, and low-fat dairy into daily meals. Nurses can guide patients in monitoring their sodium consumption, reading food labels, and making healthier choices when dining out. They can also teach patients how to prepare flavorful meals using herbs, spices, and other salt substitutes to help them adhere to the diet.

If assisting people with use of the DASH diet to manage hypertension, the nurse should expect to see systolic blood pressure dropping by about 5–11 mmHg and diastolic blood pressure dropping by about 3–6 mmHg (Natural Medicines, 2024). Nurses can consider using the modified DASH diet called MAMA-DASH, with calories and nutrition calculated for pregnancy, as this has been used safely with no reports of safety concerns (VanHorn, et al., 2018).

In addition to education, nurses have a crucial role in providing ongoing support and monitoring patients' progress. They can assess patients' dietary compliance, address challenges or obstacles they may encounter, and provide motivational counseling to help patients stay committed to their dietary goals. Nurses can collaborate with other health care professionals, such as dietitians or nutritionists, to optimize patient care and provide comprehensive guidance tailored to individual needs.

Moreover, nurses can collaborate with patients' families and caregivers, encouraging them to support dietary changes and participate in meal planning and preparation. By involving the patient's support network, nurses can create an environment conducive to long-term success in following complementary care diets.

It is also important for nurses to stay updated on the latest research and evidence regarding these diets. By staying informed, nurses can provide evidence-based information to patients, dispel myths or misunderstandings, and ensure patients are following safe and effective dietary practices.

Through education, support, and ongoing monitoring, nurses empower patients to make informed choices, ensure adherence to dietary plans, and promote overall well-being. By working collaboratively with patients, their families, and other health care professionals, nurses provide a holistic approach to managing patients' nutritional needs and promoting optimal health outcomes. Nurses are considered experts in this area and can communicate with dieticians and nutritionists on staff at their facilities with any questions regarding patients' diet, vitamins, minerals, or natural products. Interdisciplinary approaches to patient care can be extremely helpful.

Complementary nutritional interventions do not stop at diet alone. Vitamins, minerals, and natural products are sometimes referred to as nutraceuticals. We will review some of the definitions for these nutritional therapies.

Nutraceuticals: Vitamins, Minerals, and Natural Products

Nutraceuticals such as vitamins, minerals, and natural products of several kinds and also contribute to wellness and can be considered a type of complementary care. We will now discuss each of these substances separately.

Nutraceuticals

The term **nutraceutical** refers to "substances that are intended to have health benefits in addition to their basic nutritional value" (Williamson et al., 2020, p. 1227). This word emerges from a word that may be more common to nurses: nutrients. **Nutrients** are "the chemical substances supplied by food that the body needs for growth, maintenance, and repair" (Lutz et al., 2015). Nutraceuticals is an umbrella term that includes many different products, including functional foods, fortified foods, fiber, plant extracts, amino acids, vitamins, and minerals. These substances include ingredients that are recommended as safe in America (Williamson et al., 2020). Sometimes they are associated with a dosage to standardize the substance. Nutraceuticals are used extensively and are used more by certain groups of people, including older adults, those with cancer, athletes, and people who are trying to lose weight (Agbabiaka et al., 2017; Alsanad et al., 2016; Gurley et al., 2018). It is important for the nurse to have a basic understanding of vitamins, minerals, herbs, phytochemicals, prebiotics, probiotics, and other nutritional elements. People pursue use of these substances in greater amounts than are recommended to manage their health disorders, and it is important to recognize if what they are doing is safe and based on research evidence.

Vitamins

Vitamins are organic substances needed by the body in small amounts for normal metabolism, growth, and maintenance (Lutz et al., 2015). Vitamins adjust and regulate metabolic processes. They also act as coenzymes in enzymatic systems in the body. Each vitamin has a specific function in the body, and one vitamin cannot take over the functions over for a different vitamin. This makes it so important to consume all the vitamins required by the body, including both fat-soluble and water-soluble vitamins, which refer to their solubility in fat or water. The fat-soluble vitamins include A, D, E, and K. The water-soluble vitamins include C, thiamin, riboflavin, niacin, B6, folate, B12, and pantothenic acid. The amounts of vitamins needed by people of all ages have been determined. RDAs and adequate intake (AI) labels are quantified using the metric system and are in micrograms and milligrams (Lutz et al., 2015). They indicate the amount of nutrients that people should get each day. The best way to get vitamins in the right amounts is through the food that we eat, although when this is not enough people may resort to taking supplements (MedlinePlus, 2023).

Minerals

Minerals are inorganic substances that become part of the body's composition and contribute to the growth and maintenance of the body's health (Lutz et al., 2015). Minerals originate in the earth's crust and eventually become a part of the soil in which plants grow, and animals eat the minerals and humans eat both the plants and animals to absorb minerals (Lutz et al., 2015). Most minerals are multifunctional and participate in the body's regulatory and metabolic functions.

Minerals are classified as major minerals or trace minerals. The major minerals in the body are calcium, sodium and potassium, phosphorus, magnesium, sulfur, and chloride. There are 10 trace minerals: iron, iodine, fluoride, zinc, selenium, chromium, copper, manganese, cobalt, and molybdenum. There are five additional trace minerals referred to as ultra trace minerals: arsenic, boron, nickel, silicon, and vanadium (Lutz et al., 2015).

Natural Products

Let us take a moment to review some popular natural products that are in use. There are many natural products to consider, but we will review herbs, phytochemicals, probiotics, and prebiotics.

HERBS

Herbs are small, seed-bearing plants with fleshy (herbaceous) parts, rather than woody, which are useful to humans (All About Herbs, 2011). An herb may also be defined as "a plant or plant part valued for its medicinal, savory or aromatic qualities" (Bauer, 2000, p. 835).

Herbal medicines are used across the world, and use is large and steadily growing in the United States. Reasons for this increased use of herbs for health and wellness are (a) medications are seen as expensive, overprescribed, and even dangerous by some segments of the population, and (b) herbs are perceived as natural and therefore safe (Bauer, 2000). Some people are unable to afford modern-day pharmaceuticals and may take their medical treatment in their own hands. Herbs allow them to do this.

There is a problem with the sale and manufacture of herbs in the United States, and it all relates to a lack of regulation. Herbs are classified as dietary supplements since the Dietary Supplement Act of 1994 (DSHEA) was passed and the regulation of herbal therapies began to be directed by the DSHEA. Since the 1980s there has been great concern over the safety of herbs, but due to the campaign to preserve access and availability of herbs and other supplements the DSHEA allowed certain exemptions and privileges for the agents known as "dietary supplements." The DSHEA created a new definition of dietary supplements that includes "vitamins, minerals, herbs, botanicals, amino acids and other dietary substances for human use to supplement the diet" (Bauer, 2000, p. 836). Dietary supplements can be marketed without proving safety first, and the FDA is responsible for restricting herbal use only if associated health problems have been well documented (Bauer, 2000). The DSHEA does prevent manufacturers from making specific medical claims regarding a product's effectiveness (Bauer, 2000). An assumption from members of the public is that herbs are approved by the FDA, and if they are on a shelf in packaging, they are safe, but this is not the case. Herbal use in the United States has not been guaranteed to be of high quality, has great variability from brand to brand and batch to batch, or the product may not have the herb in it at all.

Aromatherapy

Aromatherapy is the "use of essential oils from plants (flower, herbs, or trees) as a complementary health approach" (National Center for Complementary and Integrative Health, 2023, para. 1). As can be seen, this therapy is closely related to herbal therapies. These essential oils are most often delivered to the client through inhalation but can also be mixed with a carrier oil and absorbed through the skin. Many essential oils are used, including bergamot, lavender, cedarwood, ginger, lemon, tea tree, geranium, chamomile, and more. Each of these essential oils have specific therapeutic purposes. Aromatherapists sometimes create a mix of specific blends of oils for specific health issues and problems.

PHYTOCHEMICALS

Phytochemicals are non-nutritive substances found in plants that contribute significantly to the flavor and color of the plants as well as the beverages derived from them (Rudzińska et al., 2023). Phytochemicals are classified into five groups: phenolics, carotenoids, organosulfur compounds, nitrogen-containing compounds, and alkaloids. Dietary phytochemicals include flavonoids, phenolic acids, phytosterols, carotenoids, and stilbenes. There is some clinical evidence to show that there is potential chemo-preventive and anticancer properties of phytochemicals (Rudzińska et al., 2023).

PROBIOTICS/PREBIOTICS

In people, the gut microbiota can be a major source of host health. Recently there has been a greater concentration on changing the composition of the gut flora with attempts made to increase helpful bacteria like Bifidobacterium and Lactobacillus that are believed to have health-promoting qualities. **Probiotics** are defined as "microbial food supplements that beneficially affect the host by improving its intestinal microbial balance," and these have been used to adjust the composition of the gut flora (Gibson & Roberfroid, 1995, p. 1401). The changes that are created by doing this are limited, so prebiotics have been added as a tool to enhance the intestinal flora. Prebiotics have been added as a tool for further improvement of the colonic microbiota. **Prebiotics** are defined as "nondigestible food ingredients that beneficially affect the host by selectively stimulating the growth and/or activity of one or a limited number of bacterial species already resident in the colon" (Gibson & Roberfroid, 1995, p. 1401). The large intestine contains the most heavily colonized area of the gastrointestinal tract. It is through the process of fermentation the colonic bacteria can create a wide range of compounds that both affect intestinal health and have other systemic influences. As of late there has been great interest in consuming both probiotics and prebiotics to enhance one's health.

Probiotics have been found to be helpful in a number of conditions, including "diarrhea, constipation, colitis, recolonization by pathogens, flatulence, gastroenteritis, gastric acidity, immunostimulant, hypercholesterolemia, hepatic encephalopathy, and carcinogenesis (Gibson & Roberfroid, 1995, p. 1405). The problem is in getting probiotics established in the large intestine, where they can adhere to the intestinal epithelium. Their chances of survival are compromised by the physical and chemical barriers in the gastrointestinal tract such as gastric acid and bile acids. They need to compete for survival with the established microbial flora of several hundred other species. Prebiotics stimulate the growth or activity of various bacteria that are already in the intestine. According to Sanders et al. (2019), "Prebiotics are substrates that are selectively utilized by host microorganisms conferring a health benefit; prebiotic effects include defense against pathogens, immune modulation, mineral absorption, bowel function, metabolic effects, and satiety (p. 606).

The use of nutritional substances to enhance health, prevent illness, and cure disease is extensive. One can expect that this area will continue to grow as new evidence of the effects of these substances on the body is discovered. Nurses and other health professionals need to keep current on the status of research evidence in this area and to remember to consult with their dietician and nutritionist colleagues for details when needed.

Discussion Questions for Your Consideration

1. Investigate the effects and precautions for one of the diets discussed in this chapter. What precautions would you give clients/ patients about this diet? What benefits have been outlined in peer-reviewed literature regarding the use of this diet for varied groups of people throughout the life span with specific health issues?
2. Choose an herb, vitamin, or supplement that you have some interest in and share with the class the actions, uses, and untoward side effects that can happen with the use of it. Consider if there are any lab studies or assessment factors that nurses can assess for and

share these with the class. Include at least three scholarly sources for your information.

3. Discuss the nurse's role in assisting patients with dietary changes for their health and wellness. Consider professional and legal issues surrounding the role requirements. Share your opinion and support your position with scholarly references.

Experiential Activities

1. Develop a teaching plan for the use of the DASH diet for the management of hypertension in a mock client. Develop at least three outcomes for learning. Outline all content of importance and the methods you would use for teaching. Discuss how the nurse would evaluate whether outcomes were met. Consider role-playing and sharing your teaching plan either online or in person.
2. Interview someone you know who is following a special diet such as a vegetarian, paleo, or DASH diet. Explore these questions:
   a. What circumstances lead you to adopting this special diet?
   b. Did a clinician guide you in the adoption of this diet? If so, what kinds of information and resources did they share with you?
   c. Have you experienced any benefits for the change in diet?
   d. Have you experienced any problems or adverse effects associated with the diet?

References

Agatston, A. (2003). *The South Beach diet.* Rodale.

Agbabiaka, T.B. Wider, B. Watson, L. K., & Goodman, C. (2017). Concurrent use of prescription drugs and herbal medicinal products in older adults: A systematic review. *Drugs and Aging, 34(*12), 891–905. https://doi.org/10.1007/s40266-017-0501-7

Arpe Gang, C. (2011, October 21) All about herbs -- botanic garden offers expansive definition of useful plants. *The Commercial Appeal*, https://www.proquest.com/docview/2595872491?accountid=13158&parentSessionId=b8SqHwXfKwtMfofNqNKeN0GXx0MDVltplPgPsODpVZA%3D&pq-origsite=summon&sourcetype=Newspapers

Alsanad, S. M., Howard, R. L., & Williamson, E. M. (2016). An assessment of the impact of herb drug combinations used by cancer patients. *BMC Complementary and Alternative Medicine*, 16, 393.

Appel, L. J., Moore, T. J., Obarzanek, E., Vollmer, W. M., Svetkey, L. P., Sacks, F. M., Bray, G. A., Vogt, T. M., Cutler, J. A., Windhauser, M. M., Lin, P. H., & Karanja, N. (1997, April). A clinical trial of the effects of dietary patterns on blood pressure. DASH Collaborative

Research Group. *New England Journal of Med*icine, 336(16), 1117–1124. https://doi.org/10.1056/NEJM199704173361601
Bauer, B. A. (2000). Herbal therapy: What a clinician needs to know to counsel patients effectively. Mayo Clinic Proceedings, 75(8), 835–841.
Bishop, F. L., Yardley, L., & Lewith, G. T. (2007). A systematic review of beliefs involved in the use of complementary and alternative medicine. *Journal of Health Psychology, 12*(6), 851–867. https://doi.org/10.1177/1359105307082447
Bliss, R. M., & Moshfegh, A. J. (2012). The Third Step—The National "What We Eat in America" Survey.
BMJ. (2023). Omega-3 fatty acid levels linked with lower risk of kidney disease. *Life Extension*, 29(6), 20.
Center for Science in the Public Interest. (2023, June). Why good nutrition is important.
Centers for Disease Control and Prevention. (2023a, April). *Heart disease*. https://www.cdc.gov/heartdisease/index.htm
Centers for Disease Control and Prevention. (2023b, June). Obesity. https://www.cdc.gov/healthyschools/obesity/index.htm
Centers for Disease Control and Prevention. (2023c, June). *Obesity facts*. https://www.cdc.gov/obesity/data/adult.html
Conlin, P. R., Chow, D., Miller, E. R., III, et al. (2000). The effect of dietary patterns on blood pressure control in hypertensive patients: Results from the Dietary Approaches to Stop Hypertension (DASH) trial. *American Journal of Hypertension*, 13, 949–955.
Dalili, D., & Bazzocchi, A. (2020). The role of body composition assessment in obesity and eating disorders. *European Journal of Radiology*, 131, 1–18.
Dinu, M., Colombini, B., Pagliai, G., et al. (2021). Effects of vegetarian versus Mediterranean diet on kidney function: Findings from the CARDIVEG study. *European Journal of Clinical Investigation, 51*(9), e13576.
Evans, J., Magee, A., Dickman, K., Sutter, R., & Sutter, C. (2017). In the community: A plant-based nutrition program. *The American Journal of Nursing, 117*(3), 56–61. https://www.jstor.org/stable/26620299
Food and Drug Administration. (2023, June). FDA 101: Dietary supplements. https://www.fda.gov/consumers/consumer-updates/fda-101-dietary-supplements
Fuchs, F.D, & Whelton, P.K. (2020, February). High blood pressure and cardiovascular disease. *Hypertension*, *75*(2), 285-292. https://doi.org/10.1161/HYPERTENSIONAHA.119.14240
Gibson, G. R., & Roberfroid, M. B. (1995). Dietary modulation of the human colonic microbiota: Introducing the concept of prebiotics. *The Journal of Nutrition, 125*(6), 1401–1412. https://doi.org/10.1093/jn/125.6.1401
Gurley, B. J., Tonsing-Carter, A., Thomas, S. L., & Fifer, E. K. (2018). Clinically relevant herb-micro nutrient interactions: When botanicals, minerals, and vitamins collide. *Advanced Nutrition, 9*(4), 5245–5325. https://doi.org/10.1093/advances/nmy029
Hoffman R. (2017). Can the paleolithic diet meet the nutritional needs of older people? *Maturitas,* 95, 63–64.
Huang, R. Y., Huang, C. C., Hu, F. B., & Chavarro, J. E. (2016). Vegetarian diets and weight reduction: A meta-analysis of randomized controlled trials. *Journal of General Internal Medicine, 31*(1), 109–116.
Huang, T., Yang, B., Zheng, J., Li, G., Wahlqvist, M. L., & Li, D. (2012). Cardiovascular disease mortality and cancer incidence in vegetarians: A meta-analysis and systematic review. Annals of Nutrition and Metabolism., 60(4), 233–240.
Jahangir, F., Daneshzad, E., Moradi, M., Maraci, M. R., Surkan, P. J., & Azadbakht, L. (2022). No association between infant growth and adherence to the dietary approaches to stop hypertension (DASH) diet in lactating women. *Nutrition and Health*. (online ahead of print), doi: 10.1177/02601060221114711.
Jew, S., AbuMweis, S. S., & Jones, P. J. (2009). Evolution of the human diet: Linking our ancestral diet to modern functional foods as a means of chronic disease prevention. *Journal of Medicinal Food*, 12(5), 925–934.

Jones-Mclean, E., Hu, J., Greene-Finestone, L. S., & de Groh, M. A. (2015). DASH dietary pattern and the risk of colorectal cancer in Canadian adults. Health Promotion and Chronic Disease Prevention in Canada., 35, 12–20.

Jonsson, T., Granfeldt, Y., Erlanson-Albertsson, C., Ahren, B., & Lindeberg, S. (2010). A paleolithic diet is more satiating per calorie than a Mediterranean-like diet in individuals with ischemic heart disease. *Nutrition and Metabolism*, 7(85).

Jonsson, T., Granfeldt, Y., Lindeberg, S., & Hallberg, A. C. (2013). Subjective satiety and other experiences of a Paleolithic diet compared to a diabetes diet in patients with type 2 diabetes. *Nutrition Journal,* 12, 105.

Kirkpatrick, C. F., Bolick, J. P., Kris-Etherton, P. M., et al. (2019). Review of current evidence and clinical recommendations on the effects of low-carbohydrate and very-low-carbohydrate (including ketogenic) diets for the management of body weight and other cardiometabolic risk factors: A scientific statement from the National Lipid Association Nutrition and Lifestyle Task Force. Journal of Clinical Lipidology, 13(5), 689–711.

Khoshbakht, Y., Moghtaderi, F., Bidaki, R., Hosseinzadeh, M., Salehi-Abargouie, A., (2021). The effect of dietary approaches to stop hypertension (DASH) diet on attention-deficit hyperactivity disorder (ADHD) symptoms: A randomized controlled clinical trial. *European Journal of Nutrition, 60* (7), 3647-3658.

Law Insider. (n.d.). Special diets definition. https://www.lawinsider.com/dictionary/special-diets

Lee, Y., & Park, K. (2017). Adherence to a vegetarian diet and diabetes risk: A systematic review and meta-analysis of observational studies. *Nutrients, 9(*6).

Levitan, E. B., Mittleman, M. A., Hakansson, N., & Wolk, A. (2007). Dietary glycemic index, dietary glycemic load, and cardiovascular disease in middle-aged and older Swedish men. *American Journal of Clinical Nutrition,* 85, 1521–1526.

Li, S., Gan, Y., Chen, M., Wang, M., Wang, X., Santos, H., Okunade,K., & Kathirgamathanby,V., (2020). Effects of the dietary approaches to stop hypertension (DASH) on pregnancy/neonatal outcomes and maternal glycemic control: A systematic review and meta-analysis of randomized clinical trials. *Complementary Therapies in Medicine, 54*, 102551. DOI: 10.1016/j.ctim.2020.102551.

Liese, A. D., Nichols, M., Sun, X., D'Agostino, R.B., & Haffner, S.M. (2009). Adherence to the DASH diet is inversely associated with incidence of type 2 diabetes: The insulin resistance atherosclerosis study. *Diabetes Care, 32*(8), 1434–1436. DOI: 10.2337/dc09-0228.

Lindeberg, S., Jonsson, T., Granfeldt, Y., Borgstrand, E., Soffman, J., Sjostrom, K., & Ahren, B. A. (2007). Paleolithic diet improves glucose tolerance more than a Mediterranean-like diet in individuals with ischaemic heart disease. *Diabetologia,* 50(9), 1795–1807.

Lutz, C., Mazur, E., & Litch, N.A. (2015). *Nutrition and Diet Therapy* (6th ed.). F.A. Davis Company.

Melina, V., Craig, W., & Levin, S. (2016). Position of the Academy of Nutrition and Dietetics: Vegetarian diets. *Journal of the Academy and Nutritional Dietetics, 116*(12), 1970–1980.

Menzel, J., Jabakhanji, A., Biemann, R., Mai, K., Abraham, K., & Weikert, C. (2020). Systematic review, and meta-analysis of the associations of vegan and vegetarian diets with inflammatory biomarkers. *Scientific Reports, 10*(1), 21736.

Mompeo, O., Berry, S. E., Spector, T. D., Menni, C., Mangina, M., Gibson, R. (2020). Differential associations between a priori diet quality scores and markers of cardiovascular health in women: Cross-sectional analyses from Twin Suk. *British Journal of Nutrition*, 1–11. DOI: 10.1017/S000711452000495X

Mozaffarian, D., & Wu, J. (2011). Omega-3 fatty acids and cardiovascular disease. *Journal of the American College of Cardiology, 58*(20), 2047–2067. https://doi.org/10.1016/j.jacc.2011.06.063

Murdaugh, C. L., Parsons, M. A., & Pender, N. J. (2019). *Health promotion in nursing practice.* Pearson.

National Cancer Institute (2023, June). Definition of vitamin. https://www.cancer.gov/publications/dictionaries/cancer-terms/def/vitamin
National Center for Complementary and Integrative Health. (2023, September). Aromatherapy. https://www.nccih.nih.gov/health/aromatherapy
Natural Medicines. (2023, March). Mediterranean Diet [monograph]. http://naturalmedicines.therapeutic research.com.
Natural Medicines. (2022, December). Vegetarian Diet. [monograph]. http://natural medicines.therapeutic research.com.
Natural Medicines. (2021, December). Paleo Diet. [monograph]. http://naturalmedicines.therapeutic research.com.
Natural Medicines (2024, March). Dash Diet [monograph]. http://naturalmedicines.therapeuticresearch.com
O'Keefe, J. H., Jr., & Cordain, L. (2004). Cardiovascular disease resulting from a diet and lifestyle at odds with our Paleolithic genome: How to become a 21st-century hunter-gatherer. *Mayo Clinical Practice, 79*(1), 101–108.
Otten, J., Ryberg, M., Mellberg, C., et al. (2019). Postprandial levels of GLP-1, GIP, and glucagon after 2 years of weight loss with a Paleolithic diet: A randomized controlled trial in healthy obese women. *European Journal of Endocrinology.*, 180(6), 417–427.
Pattar, S., Shetty, P., & Shetty, G. B. (2023). Impact of vegetarian diet on health outcomes in male individuals: A comparative study. *Advances in Integrative Medicine*, 10, 1–7.
Rudzińska, A., Juchaniuk, P., Oberda, J., Wiśniewska, J., Wojdan, W., Szklener, K., & Mańdziuk, S. (2023). Phytochemicals in cancer treatment and cancer prevention—Review on epidemiological data and clinical trials. *Nutrients, 15*(8), 1896. https://doi.org/10.3390/nu15081896
Sanders, M. E., Merenstein, D. J., Reid, G., Gibson, G. R., & Rastall, R. A., (2019, October). Probiotics And prebiotics in intestinal health and disease: From biology to the clinic. *Nature Reviews/ Gastroenterology and Hepatology,* 16, 605–616.
Salehi-Abargouei, A., Maghsoudi, Z., Shirani, F., & Azadbakht, L. (2013). Effects of dietary approaches to stop hypertension (DASH)-style diet on fatal or nonfatal cardiovascular diseases—incidence: Systematic review and meta-analysis on observational prospective studies. *Nutrition, 29*, 611–618.
Saneei, P., Salehi-Abargouei, A., Esmaillzadeh, A., & Azadbakht, L. (2014). Influence of dietary approaches to stop hypertension (DASH) diet on blood pressure: A systematic review and meta-analysis on randomized controlled trials. *Nutrition, Metabolism and Cardiovascular Diseases, 24,* 1253–1261
Soltani, S., Shirani, F., Chitsazi, M. J., & Salehi-Abargouei, A. (2016). The effect of dietary approaches to stop hypertension (DASH) diet on weight and body composition in adults: A systematic review and meta- analysis of randomized controlled clinical trials. *Obesity Review, 17,* 442–454.
Svetkey, L. P., Simons-Morton, D., Vollmer, W. M., Appel, L.J., Conlin, P.R., Ryan, D.H., Ard, J., & Kennedy, B.M. (1999). Effects of dietary patterns on blood pressure: Subgroup analysis of the Dietary Approaches to Stop Hypertension (DASH) randomized clinical trial. *Archives of Internal Medicine,159*, 285–293. View abstract.
Tan, C., Zhao, Y., & Wang, S. (2019). Is a vegetarian diet safe to follow during pregnancy? A systematic review and meta-analysis of observational studies. *Critical Reviews in Food Science and Nutrition, 59*(16), 2586–2596.
Van Horn, L., Carson, J. S., Appel, L. J., Burke, L. E., Economos, C., Karmally, W., Lancaster, K., Lichtenstein, A. H., Johnson, R. K., Thomas, R. J., Vos, M., Wylie-Rosett, J., & Kris-Etherton, P. (2016). Recommended dietary pattern to achieve adherence to the American Heart Association/American College of Cardiology (AHA/ACC) guidelines. *Circulation, 134*(22), e505–e529. https://doi.org/10.1161/CIR.0000000000000462
Van Horn, L., Peaceman, A., Kwasny, M., Vincent, E., Fought, A., Josefson, J., Spring, B., Neff, L.M., & Gernhofer, N. (2018). Dietary approaches to stop hypertension diet and activity to limit gestational weight: Maternal Offspring Metabolic Family Intervention

Trial, a technology enhanced randomized trial. *American Journal of Preventative Medicine.*, 55(5), 603–614.
Viguiliouk, E., Kendall, C. W., Kahleová, H., Rahelic, D., Salas-Salvoda, J., Choo, V.L., Blanco Mejias, S., Stewardt, S.E., Leiter, L.A., Jenkins, D.J., & Sievenpiper, J.L. (2018). Effect of vegetarian dietary patterns on cardiometabolic risk factors in diabetes: A systematic review and meta-analysis of randomized controlled trials. *Clinical Nutrition*, Jun;38(3):1133-1145. doi: 10.1016/j.clnu.2018.05.032.
Wang, T., Heianza, Y., Sun, D., Huang, T., Ma, W., Rimm, E. B., Manson, J.E., Hu, F.B., Willett, W.C, & Qi, L.(2018). Improving adherence to healthy dietary patterns, genetic risk, and long-term weight gain: Gene-diet interaction analysis in two prospective cohort studies. British Medical Journal, 360, k693. DOI: 10.1136/bmj.j5644
Williamson, E. M., Xinmin, L., & Izzo, A. A. (2020). Trends in nurse, pharmacology, and clinical applications of emerging herbal nutraceuticals. *British Journal of Pharmacology*, 177, 1227–1240.

Credits

Fig. 3.1: Copyright © 2019 Depositphotos/bit245.
Fig. 3.2: USDA, https://commons.wikimedia.org/wiki/File:USDA_MyPlate_green.svg, U.S. Department of Agriculture, 2011.
Fig. 3.3: Copyright © 2015 Depositphotos/petitelili.

CHAPTER 4

Physical Therapies

> "To keep the body in good health is a duty...otherwise we shall not be able to keep the mind strong and clear."
>
> —BUDDHA

Objectives

This chapter will enable the reader to do the following:

1. Identify select complementary therapies that work in the physical domain and are used to promote optimum health and care for common health disorders.
2. Discuss the theoretical rationale for the mode of action of select physical therapies.
3. Compare and contrast physical therapies, including chiropractic/osteopathic manipulation, massage therapy, light stimulation, electrical stimulation, color therapy, and heat/cold therapy.
4. Discuss common uses for selecting physical therapies in people.
5. Describe evidence-based effects of various physical therapies.
6. Discuss potential adverse effects of physical therapies on people.
7. Describe the role of the nurse and other health care providers in guiding patients regarding their use of select physical therapies.
8. Discuss the types of specialized education required and guidelines for those who wish to help people with using the select physical therapies.

Key Terms

Chiropractic: "A licensed health care profession that emphasizes the body's ability to heal itself. Treatment typically involves manual therapy, often including spinal manipulation. Other forms of treatment, such as exercise and nutritional counseling, may be used as well" (National Center for Complementary and Integrative Health, 2023, para. 1).

Massage therapy: Involves the manipulation of soft tissues in the body, including muscles, tendons, and ligaments.

Light therapy: "Also known as phototherapy involves exposing the skin to specific wavelengths of light to help with a variety of conditions" (Natural Medicines, 2023, March)

Color therapy: Also known as chromotherapy, the use of color for therapeutic purposes (Natural Medicines, 2023).

Electrotherapy: Includes several interventions that use electricity for therapeutic reasons.

Heat and cold therapies: Involve the application of temperature to affected areas of the body for therapeutic purposes.

Introduction

In this chapter we will review select complementary therapies that are believed to work in a physical way in the body and are used for complementary and integrative care. Complementary and alternative therapies encompass a wide range of practices that aim to promote healing, improve well-being, or address health concerns. While many therapies focus on the mind and spirit, there are several therapies that are believed to have primarily a physical impact on the body. We will focus on chiropractic/osteopathic manipulation, massage therapy, light stimulation, electrotherapy, and heat/cold therapy. For each of these therapy types we will address the mode of actions, the common uses, the potential benefits, the potential adverse effects, and the role of the nurse and other health care professionals as a part of interdisciplinary care in guiding patients in their use and any special education that one needs to provide such a therapy.

Chiropractic Therapy

Chiropractic and osteopathy emerged in folk traditions involving "bone setting." Each of these therapies originated in the United States (Vickers & Zollman, 1999). The founders of each therapy met up with Daniel D. Palmer, the founder of chiropractic care, and with Taylor Still, the founder of osteopathy. Later, each man set up his own school. The therapies are very similar, and they tend to use common terminology and scholarly sources (Vickers & Zollman, 1999). Since they are similar, we will limit our discussion to the outline of chiropractic therapy.

Chiropractic therapy emphasizes the body's ability to heal itself. Its use has been increasing in different countries over the last decades and addresses neuromuscular disorders and their influence on whole body health (Salehi et al., 2015). The WHO's (2005) definition of chiropractic care is "a healthcare profession concerned with the diagnosis, treatment and prevention of disorders of the neuromusculoskeletal system, and the effects of these disorders on health" (as cited in Salehi et al., 2015). Treatment typically involves manual therapy, often including spinal manipulation. Other forms of treatment, such as exercise and nutritional counseling, may be used as well (National Center for Complementary and Integrative Health, 2023). Chiropractic therapy focuses particularly on the spine to improve overall health. It involves manual manipulation of the spine to align the vertebrae, relieve pain, and restore proper nerve function.

Care from a chiropractor might include adjustments to realign joints, exercises and stretching, soft tissue therapy, joint taping/bracing for support of weakened areas, and referrals to other therapists or providers of care (Cleveland Clinic, 2023).

Therapeutic Uses of Chiropractic Therapy

Chiropractors use hands-on techniques to manipulate and adjust the body, aiming to improve alignment, reduce pain, and enhance the body's natural healing abilities. The most common reasons for a chiropractic adjustment include back pain, neck pain, muscular pain, and headaches (Cleveland Clinic, 2023).

Evidence-Based Effects of Chiropractic Therapy

Evidence is growing, and some effectiveness of chiropractic care has been revealed. In one study that sought to evaluate the effectiveness of chiropractic in the treatment of different diseases, a systematic review was completed of 11 chiropractic systematic reviews focusing on the effectiveness of chiropractic treatment. The results revealed that chiropractic treatment improves neck pain, shoulder and neck trigger points, and sport injuries. The same study found that regarding asthma, infant colic, autism spectrum disorder, gastrointestinal problems, fibromyalgia, back pain, and carpal tunnel syndrome, no conclusive scientific evidence for treatment effectiveness was apparent. More study was recommended by this group of researchers (Salehi et al., 2015).

Potential Adverse Effects and Concerns

Chiropractic care, like any form of medical treatment, may have potential adverse effects. About 50% of patients who have received spinal manipulative therapy (SMT) have experienced some type of benign adverse event (BAE), which was usually benign and temporary (Fuanabashi et al., 2020). It is crucial to note that BAEs are uncommon, but they should not be disregarded. The effects need to be addressed to improve quality of care and the experience of the patient. In one 11-question survey that was administered by exploring beliefs, perceptions, and practices regarding BAEs after SMT and strategies to address them, 39 clinicians and 203 patients were surveyed. For the patients, 55% reported experiencing some BAE after SMT, which involved mostly pain/soreness, headache, and stiffness (Funabashi et al., 2020). Clinicians reported trying a mitigation strategy (61.5%) to manage these BAEs. These strategies included soft tissue therapy (75%), stretching (62.5%), and icing (45.8%). All 24 clinicians reported having some success in mitigating these benign BAEs post-SMT (Funabashi et al., 2020). More research is needed to examine the effects both positive and negative of chiropractic interventions, but it is helpful to know that BAEs are possible and can be mitigated. Patients should be informed of this possibility before pursuing chiropractic care.

Nurse Guidance for Use of Chiropractic Therapy

The role of a nurse in guiding and teaching patients about chiropractic care is to provide valuable information and support. Nurses can educate patients about the principles of chiropractic care, explaining how it focuses on the spine and nervous system to improve overall health. They can discuss the benefits and potential risks of chiropractic adjustments, helping patients make informed decisions. Nurses can also address any concerns or misconceptions patients may have, ensuring they have a clear understanding of what to expect during chiropractic treatments. By offering guidance and education, nurses empower patients to actively participate in their chiropractic care journey.

Types of Special Education Required

To become a chiropractor, individuals must complete extensive educational requirements. The educational path typically starts with a bachelor's degree, which can be in a variety of fields, but commonly in biology, chemistry, or a related science discipline. After obtaining a bachelor's degree, aspiring chiropractors must then attend a chiropractic college or university accredited by the Council on Chiropractic Education (National Center for Complementary and Integrative Health, 2023).

Chiropractic programs usually span 4 years of full-time study, combining classroom instruction, laboratory work, and clinical experience. During this time, students learn about anatomy, physiology, pathology, diagnostic imaging, chiropractic techniques, and patient care. They also gain practical experience through internships and clinical rotations under the supervision of licensed chiropractors.

Upon graduation, individuals must pass the standardized National Board of Chiropractic Examinations (NBCE) to become licensed practitioners. Additional state-specific requirements may also exist, such as jurisprudence exams or practical exams (National Center for Complementary and Integrative Health, Chiropractic in Depth, 2023). Continuing education is essential for chiropractors to maintain their licenses and stay abreast of the latest advancements in the field. Many states require chiropractors to complete a certain number of continuing education credits to renew their licenses periodically.

Massage Therapy

Massage therapy involves the manipulation of soft tissues in the body, including muscles, tendons, and ligaments. It can relieve anxiety, depression, and pain (Moyer et al., 2010). Research suggests that massage therapy may have physiological effects such as increased blood flow, improved immune function, and reduced levels of stress hormones (Moyer et al., 2011). Massage therapy has been shown to stimulate the activation of the parasympathetic nervous system (Diego & Field, 2009). It has also been asserted that the sympathetic nervous systems are suppressed through stimulation of skin receptors innervated by vagal fibres (Delaney et al., 2002; Diego & Field, 2009). This leads to a decrease in the vital signs: pulse, blood pressure, and respiratory rate (Vahedian-Aximi, et al., 2014). Desirable psychological effects such as feelings of increased comfort and a reduction in anxiety occur (Cutshall et al., 2010). There are several types of therapeutic massage, each with its own unique techniques and benefits (Table 4.1).

Table 4.1 The Most Common Types of Massage

Massage Type	Description
Swedish massage	Involves the use of long, gliding strokes, kneading, and circular movements on the superficial layers of muscles. It is known for promoting relaxation, reducing muscle tension, and improving circulation.
Deep tissue massage	This type of massage targets deeper layers of muscle and connective tissue to alleviate chronic muscle tension and adhesion. The therapist uses slow, firm strokes and deep pressure to reach underlying muscles and fascia.
Sports massage	Specifically designed for athletes, sports massage aims to enhance athletic performance, prevent injuries, and promote recovery. It combines various techniques to address specific muscle groups and areas of tension.
Trigger point therapy	This type of massage focuses on releasing trigger points, which are tight knots in the muscles that can cause referred pain in other parts of the body. The therapist applies pressure to these points to relieve pain and restore normal muscle function.
Shiatsu massage	Originating from Japan, shiatsu massage involves applying rhythmic pressure on specific points along the body's meridians (energy pathways). It aims to balance the body's energy flow and promote overall well-being.

Table 4.1 The Most Common Types of Massage

Thai massage	Based on traditional Thai medicine, this massage incorporates stretching, acupressure, and yoga-like movements. The therapist uses their hands, knees, legs, and feet to apply pressure and facilitate stretching to improve flexibility and energy flow.
Hot stone massage	Smooth, heated stones are used in combination with traditional massage techniques to relax muscles and promote deep relaxation. The heat from the stones helps to increase blood flow and relieve tension.
Prenatal massage	Tailored for pregnant women, prenatal massage focuses on addressing the unique needs and discomforts associated with pregnancy. It helps relieve lower back pain, reduces swelling, and promotes relaxation.

It is important to note that therapists may integrate multiple techniques in their sessions, customizing the treatment based on the client's needs and preferences. Consulting with a qualified massage therapist can help determine the best type of massage for specific concerns.

Therapeutic Uses of Massage Therapy

Massage therapy is used for pain management, stress reduction, relaxation, injury rehabilitation, mental health improvement, and sports performance enhancement. It promotes circulation, reduces muscle tension, enhances well-being, and can be beneficial for a variety of physical and emotional conditions.

Evidence-Based Effects of Massage Therapy

Massage therapy has been shown to be helpful in the reduction of several types of pain: low-back pain, neck and shoulder pain, pain from osteoarthritis of the knee, and headaches (National Center for Complementary and Integrative Health, 2023).

In one study involving a systematic review of the impact of massage on critically ill patients, researchers found that massage implementation in critical care can have a positive effect on multiple patient outcomes, including improvement in hemodynamic measures, decreased pain intensity, decreased anxiety, and enhanced sleep (Jagan et al., 2019). Researchers investigated the impact of massage therapy on those with Parkinson's disease in a systematic review of 12 studies (Angelopoulou et al., 2020). What they found was massage-induced relaxation in most cases, which was associated with biological measures of urine stress hormones. They also discovered nonmotor symptoms, including sleep disturbances, pain, fatigue, anxiety, and symptoms of depression were improved with massage.

In a systematic review and meta-analysis to examine the effect massage therapy on both pain and anxiety in persons with burns it was found that massage therapy significantly reduced the intensity of anxiety and the intensity of pain in burn patients (Miri et al., 2023). Researchers found in a systematic review and meta-analysis that compared to usual care, massage therapy when combined with passive mobilizations showed an improvement in weight gain and a reduction in length of hospitalization in preterm infants (Molla-Casanova et al., 2023). These are some of the many positive effects of massage.

Potential Adverse Effects and Concerns

When it comes to massage therapy, there are several potential adverse effects to consider. It is important to note that these effects are rare, and most people experience positive outcomes from massage. However, here are some potential adverse effects that have been reported in certain cases:

- Soreness and discomfort: Deep tissue or intense massages can cause temporary soreness and discomfort, especially if it is your first massage or if the therapist uses strong pressure. However, this typically subsides within a couple of days.
- Bruising or skin irritation: Overly aggressive or rough massages may result in bruising or skin irritation. This can occur when excessive pressure is applied or when the therapist does not use enough lubrication. Individuals with sensitive or fragile skin may be more prone to experiencing this.
- Aggravation of existing conditions: In some cases, massage therapy can worsen certain conditions. For example, if you have a recent injury, infectious skin condition, or circulatory disorders

like deep vein thrombosis, the wrong type of massage or improper technique can potentially exacerbate these conditions.
- Allergic reactions: Some individuals may have allergic reactions to the oils, lotions, or other substances used during the massage. If you have known allergies or sensitivities, it is essential to inform your therapist beforehand to ensure they avoid using any potentially allergic substances.
- Psychological response: In rare cases, individuals may experience emotional or psychological reactions during or after a massage. Feelings of sadness, anxiety, or even euphoria can occur. This is thought to be related to the release of certain neurotransmitters and hormones triggered by massage.

The risk of harmful effects from massage therapy appears to be low. However, there have been rare reports of serious side effects, such as a blood clot, nerve injury, or bone fracture. Some of the reported cases have involved vigorous types of massage, such as deep tissue massage, or patients who might be at increased risk of injury, such as elderly people (National Center for Complementary and Integrative Therapies, 2023).

It is important to remember that most people experience only positive outcomes and feel relaxed and rejuvenated after a massage. However, to minimize the risks and maximize the benefits, it is recommended to consult with a qualified massage therapist, communicate any existing health conditions or concerns, and ensure that the therapist is skilled, reputable, and licensed.

Nurse Guidance for Use of Massage Therapy

Nurses can provide valuable guidance to patients who are interested in massage therapy. Nurses can inform patients about the potential benefits of massage therapy, such as stress reduction, pain relief, improved circulation, enhanced relaxation, and even improved immune function. They can emphasize that massage therapy is considered safe and may complement conventional medical treatments.

Nurses can help patients identify their goals for seeking massage therapy. Whether it is pain management, relaxation, stress reduction, or addressing specific health conditions, understanding the patient's goals can help determine the type of massage therapy that would be most suitable. Nurses can guide patients on locating qualified and licensed massage therapists. They can provide information about professional associations (e.g., American Massage Therapy Association), online directories, or local resources that list reputable therapists.

Patients should be encouraged to communicate openly with their massage therapist. They should discuss any existing health conditions, allergies, or medications they are taking. Open communication allows the therapist to tailor the massage to the patient's specific needs and avoid any potential adverse effects.

Nurses can inform patients about potential precautions to consider. For example, patients with certain conditions, such as fractures, burns, infectious skin diseases, or recent surgeries, may require adjustments or specific techniques. Patients with high blood pressure should be careful with deep pressure massages.

Jagan et al. (2019) suggested that when working in intensive care environments that various elements need to be properly considered, specifically in the planning and implementation phase, such as the amount of pressure used and its impact on neurotransmission, body areas massaged, the number of repetitions used, and the necessity of receiving proper training and education on the massage techniques used, as well as full consideration of both patient preferences and family preferences when the patient is unable to speak for themselves (Jagan et al., 2019).

Nurses can remind patients to assess the effectiveness of the massage therapy sessions and provide feedback to their therapist. If the patient does not experience the desired outcomes or if any adverse effects occur, they should consult with the therapist and, if necessary, their health care provider.

It is important to note that nurses should consult reliable sources and research studies when providing guidance to patients. They can refer to reputable health care websites, professional associations, or relevant scientific literature to ensure the information they share is evidence-based and up-to-date.

Types of Special Education Required

In the United States, the education requirements for massage therapists vary by state. The minimum requirement is completion of a postsecondary program with a curriculum focused on massage therapy. These programs typically include coursework in anatomy, physiology, kinesiology, ethics, and various massage techniques. In some states, aspiring massage therapists may also need to pass a licensing exam or meet additional requirements. Additional education and certifications can be pursued to specialize in specific techniques or modalities. In some states massage therapy is regulated (45 states and the District of Columbia), and massage therapists must get a license or certification before practicing massage (National Center for Complementary and Integrative Health, 2023). State regulations typically require graduation from an approved program and passing an examination.

Massage therapists may obtain certification from the National Certification Board for Therapeutic Massage & Bodywork. To be certified, the applicant must meet educational requirements, undergo a background check, and then pass an examination (National Center for Complementary and Integrative Health, 2023). It is important to note that specific education requirements can vary, so it is advisable to check the regulations of the state where one intends to practice.

Light Stimulation

Light therapy, "also known as phototherapy, involves exposing the skin to specific wavelengths of light in order to help with a variety of conditions" (Natural Medicines, 2023). It can involve exposure to natural sunlight or involve the use of artificial light sources. Light therapy can be administered by using light-emitting diodes (LEDs), fluorescent lamps, lasers, dichroic lamps, or very bright full-spectrum light (Natural Medicines, 2023). Light therapy is commonly used to treat seasonal affective disorder (SAD), a type of depression that occurs during certain times of the year and hyperbilirubinemia (Horn, 2019).

Light therapy works by regulating circadian rhythms and influencing serotonin levels, which can improve mood and alleviate depressive symptoms (Terman et al., 1989). Many distinct types of light therapy devices have been invented using different light sources (Natural Medicines, 2023). Some light sources used are blue, fluorescent tubes, light-emitting diode (LED) sources, halogen, and fiber-optic light. In some cases, light therapy is given directly, and in others through concentrators and filters. Light therapy may be given to the entire body or to a specific area (spot treatment). Devices such as light boxes, with high-intensity florescent lights, may be used, as is seen with treatment for mood and sleep disorders. Treatments are delivered to dermatologists' offices, health centers, or light therapy clinics. Home devices for distinct types of light therapy are also available for purchase and home use (Natural Medicines, 2023; see Figure 4.1).

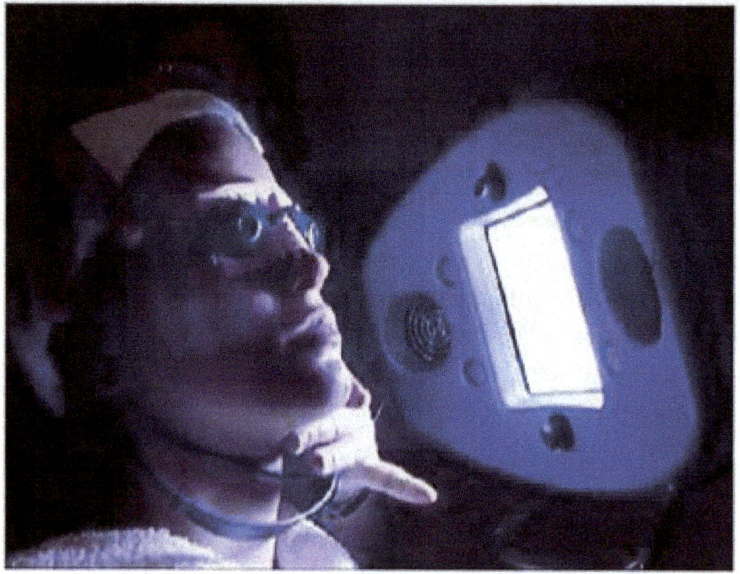

Figure 4.1 Blue light acne phototherapy using the iClear by Curelight Ltd.

Therapeutic Uses of Light Stimulation

Light therapy has shown promise in treating sleep disorders, nonseasonal depression, hyperbilirubinemia, and certain skin conditions such as psoriasis. Its uses range from the treatment of seasonal affective disorder (SAD) and depression to sleep disorders, skin conditions like psoriasis and eczema, and jet lag. Light therapy works by mimicking natural sunlight and affecting the production of certain hormones and neurotransmitters in the body. While many studies demonstrate its effectiveness, it is important to consult a health care professional before using light therapy. Their guidance can ensure proper treatment and minimize potential risks.

Evidence-Based Effects of Light Stimulation

Light therapy has been shown to have treatment effects in a wide array of clinical disorders. Before the 1950s neonatal jaundice was a frequent problem and often lead to the death of premature infants. A British nurse by the name of Sister Jean Ward believed that fresh air and sunshine benefited frailer infants, and she serendipitously discovered that taking infants who were premature out into the sun eradicated their jaundice (Daily Nurse, 2023). Sister Jean Ward's observations lead the way to the use of phototherapy treatments that are still used today to combat hyperbilirubinemia in infants. Phototherapy is now given with specialized devices on neonatal units that deliver a certain wavelength of light for hyperbilirubinemia (Horn, 2019). Light therapy was used as a part of treatment of children and others while in the care of nurses at health centers like the Lister Trust Wards of Vienna in 1920–1922.

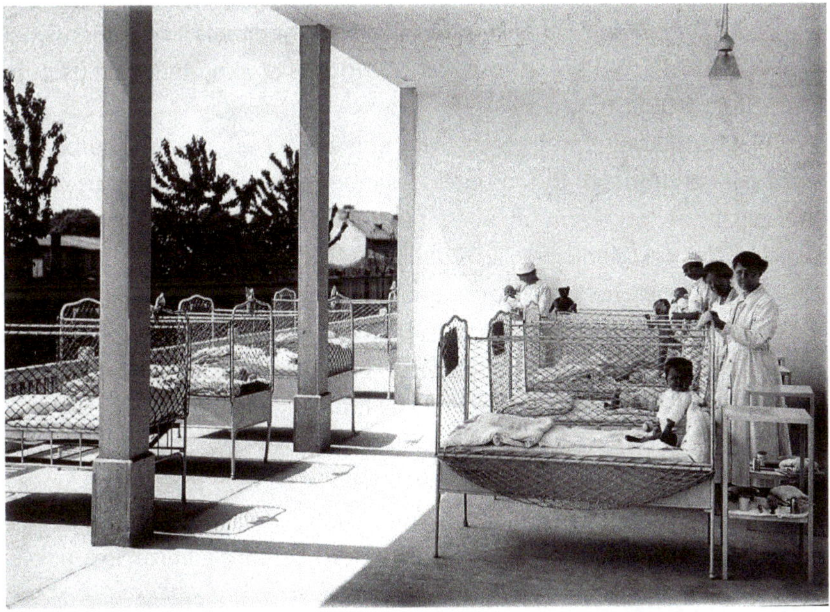

Figure 4.2 Children receiving sun treatment in the veranda of the Lister Trust Wards of Vienna in the garden of the University Kinderklinic, Vienna, 1920–1922.

Light therapy has been shown to help with skin disorders such as the scaly, itchy, skin of psoriasis using ultraviolent B (UVB) and ultraviolet A (UVA) light, eczema with UVB and UVA, cold sores with a special lighting device, scleroderma with UVA, and vitiligo and itching with the UVB light (Natural Medicines, 2023). Psychological issues and mood disorders also respond to light therapy with bipolar depression, sleep–wake cycle disturbances such as insomnia, SAD, and depression all responding (Chang et al., 2018; Natural Medicines, 2023; Terman et al., 1989).

Potential Adverse Effects and Concerns

Light therapy, while considered safe, can have some adverse effects. Some clients might report ocular complaints, as in one systematic review in which complaints of discomfort and vision problems were reported in 0% to 45% of participants in studies of light therapy (Brouwer et al., 2017). Skin reactions like redness, itching, or rash are possible with certain types of light therapy. Light therapy, when given for skin conditions, can cause polymorphic light eruption, which is a type of rash. Persons with scleroderma, granuloma annulare, and skin conditions that cause small scaling raised spots are at greatest risk for developing this rash (Natural Medicines, 2023).

Light therapy can interact with some medications and herbs. For example, people on the drug psoralen (PUVA) should not use light therapy in the long-term because it can increase their risk for squamous cancer (Natural Medicines, 2023). Some medications might make the skin more sensitive to sunlight, leading to blistering, rashes, and other side effects. Giving light therapy to persons using certain herbs such as bishop's weed, khella, St. John's wort, and chlorophyll are at increased risk for rashes and other side effects (Natural Medicines, 2023).

It is important to consult a health care professional before starting light therapy, especially if you have preexisting eye conditions or are taking medications that can interact with light. Always follow the recommended guidelines and duration of use to minimize the risk of adverse effects.

Nurse Guidance for Use of Light Therapy

The nurse plays a crucial role in assisting patients undergoing light therapy. They can educate patients about the treatment, including its purpose, benefits, and potential side effects. Nurses can also assess patients for any contraindications or precautions that may affect the use of light therapy. They monitor patients' progress, ensure adherence to treatment schedules, and address any concerns or questions. Additionally, nurses can provide emotional support and help patients manage any discomfort or adverse effects that may arise. Collaboration with other health care team members is important to facilitate comprehensive care for patients undergoing light therapy.

Types of Special Education Required

It is important that one learns about the special type of light therapy they intend to get treatment with. Some light therapy is available for the public to use without any educational training or degree, but patients should be assured that they are following the device's directions for use. It may be wise to start out with small doses of light therapy so that one can assess the effects initially before starting a full treatment. If the nurse is delivering light therapy, it is important to know what equipment you are using and how to use it. As always, it is important to assess continually at the start, during, and following treatment with any light device. Assessing clients at pretreatment and posttreatment gives the nurse or clinician valuable data pertaining to the light therapies effectiveness as well as assisting in identifying a complication. Certifications in light therapy are available to assist with gaining the knowledge that is required to use light therapy.

Color Therapy

Color therapy, also known as chromotherapy, "is the use of color for therapeutic purposes" (Natural Medicines, 2020). This therapy is based on the belief that colors have specific vibrational frequencies that can affect our physical, mental, and emotional states. Color therapy is sometimes provided in the form of light. Researchers have suggested that color therapy is "a method of treatment that uses the visible spectrum (colors) of electromagnetic radiation to cure diseases" (Azemi et al., 2018).

Color and light therapy have their roots in ancient medicine (Roseman-Halsband, 2018).

Color therapists believe that each color corresponds to a specific energy center or chakra in our body and that by using the appropriate colors, we can stimulate or calm these energy centers, thus promoting healing. Different colors are associated with different qualities and emotions. For example, red is believed to stimulate energy and vitality, while blue is associated with calmness and relaxation (Gupta, 2021).

Color therapy can be applied in several ways. One common practice is through colored light therapy, in which colored lights are shone onto specific parts of the body or the entire body to create a healing effect. Another technique involves using colored crystals or gemstones, as they are thought to emit specific vibrational frequencies.

Practitioners of color therapy may also recommend incorporating specific colors into our everyday lives, such as wearing certain colored clothing, painting our living spaces with specific hues, or even eating foods that are naturally rich in particular colors. Some of the other ways that color therapy is delivered are through solarized water; massaging with color-saturated oils; eating colored foods; directing the client to wear certain colors; having the client focus on an object that is saturated with a certain color such a colored paper, cloth, or glass; or color breathing in which the individual is taken through a guided meditation when they imagine breathing in and out various colors.

In the 1920s light therapies were used by physicians, and many different therapeutic devices for the delivery of color evolved. These included electric light baths and the use of wooden cabinets lit up with incandescent lamps that were especially helpful for those with arthritis (Roseman-Halsband, 2018).

Most individuals are aware of how assorted colors may affect them, but the use of color is theorized as having effects beyond those involving psychological influence. For example, one group of researchers studied the impact of green light exposure, also referred to as green light–emitting diode (GLED) in a color-blind patient demonstrating a reduction in severity of headache pain but not frequency, as had been seen in the patient's previous research. The researchers were trying to explore the underlying mechanisms of this type of color therapy. They hypothesized that GLED-induced analgesia is dependent on M-cone photo-recognition, and in the color-blind client less analgesia occurred because of activation of both M-cones (antinociceptive) and L-cones (proprioceptive), with in turn less pronounced improvements in both the frequency of his headache pain and quality of life. These researchers proposed that "the activation of only M-cones in normal vision patients and the activation of both M-cones and L-cones in this protanomalous (color blind) subject provided an explanation for the differences in response to GLED in these two patient populations" (Cheng et al., 2022, p. 6).

Carl Loeb, MD, in his book Specific Light Therapy, used the terms "light frequencies," "wavelengths," or "spectral band" and asserted that "color is synonymous with chemistry, which can be utilized in the body to create energy and function activity" (Loeb, 1927, as cited in Roseman-Halsband, 2018, p. 123). Loeb believed that the most essential element for the delivery of colored light therapy was the absorption of energy by the body when the cellular structure could be changed. He studied the use of colored light as therapy for 18 years of his life (Roseman-Halsband, 2018).

Other therapists claim to use different lights in the form of color to maintain an energy that is lacking from the individual. The element that is lacking could be physical, emotional, spiritual, or mental, and various colors provide different energies. Different colors are then used to treat different illnesses or conditions. For example, blue or purple light is believed to have calming and anti-inflammatory effects, and red is exciting, which could be overstimulating in the client who is not in need of this influence (Gupta, 1068). Chakras were discussed earlier in this text as energy centers in the body in our discussion of Indian philosophy as a basis for some complementary therapies. It is interesting to note that each chakra is associated with different colors, and the colors are believed to have different functions on the body (Figure 4.3).

Root Chakra – Physical Well Being

Use **red** to restore your passion to live. Red transforms anger and frustration into positive power to reclaim your free existence on earth, it helps grounding and accepting your physical being.

Red helps to:

- energize yourself physically
- overcome fear
- develop morning sickness
- stimulate appetite

Essential Oils and Incense

Cedar, Cinnamon, Clove, Sage, Sandalwood, Yang Ylang.

Herbs and Supplements

Ginseng, Golden Seal, Valerian

Proteins, Root Vegetables

Beets, Cayenne Pepper, Cherries, Radishes, Red Pepper, Strawberries, Tomatoes, Watermelon.

Gemstones

Agate, Bloodstone, Garnet, Hematite, Red Tiger's Eye, Ruby

Affirmation

I deserve my own place to exist in freedom.

Sacral Chakra – Creativity and Playfulness

Use **orange** to find creative solutions and happiness. Orange releases compulsive behavior, inhibitions, dissatisfaction and self-doubt. It removes reluctance to live by easing anxiety on the physical (sexual) level.

Orange helps to:

- enjoy sexual activity
- raise ambition
- ease anxiety and low self esteem

Essential Oils and Incense

Angelica, Gardenia, Lemon Grass, Melissa, Orange

Herbs and Supplements

Grape Seed, Raspberry, Uva Ursi

Food

Carrots, Oranges, Peaches, Pumpkins, Yams

Gemstones

Carnelian, Copper, Coral, Moonstone

Affirmation

I am allowed to create my own space, my own life.

Solar Plexus – Free Will, Clear Mind

Use **yellow** to restore mental clarity and free will. Yellow helps you to follow instinct and feelings, it revitalizes you mentally as well as physically by transforming mental and physical resistance and memory problems.

Yellow helps to:

- overcome digestive disorders
- overcome memory problems
- overcome fatigue

Essential Oils and Incense

Bergamot, Grapefruit, Fennel, Lemon, Rosemary

Herbs and Supplements

Ginger, Goldenseal, Lemon Balm, Milk Thistle

Food

Bananas, Corn, Eggs, Grapefruit, Lemons, Melons, Yellow Vegetables, Pineapples, Yellow Peppers

Gemstones

Amber, Citrine, Gold, Topaz, Yellow Sapphire

Affirmation

I allow myself to be strong, and to stand up for myself.

Heart Chakra – Harmony, Balance, Love	Throat Chakra – Function in Life, Vocation	Brow Chakra – Inspiration / Intelligence
Use **green** to live in the 'Here and Now'. Green balances your yin/yang (male and female) character traits, it harmonizes your body/ spirit and frees you to live your future from limitations of the past. Green helps to: • calm down from panic or anxiety • free yourself from jealousy • transform disharmony in relationships to a state of balance **Essential Oils and Incense** Cedarwood, Eucalyptus, Pine **Herbs and Supplements** Comfrey, Hyssop, Pine, Sage **Food** Green Vegetables, Avocados, Artichokes, Beans, Broccoli, Brussels Sprouts, Cabbage, Cucumber, Green Salads, Peas, and other Green Vegetables **Gemstones** Aventurine, Emerald, Jade, Malachite, Peridot **Affirmation** I allow myself to feel. My emotions are valid and right.	Use **blue** to restore your functioning at home and work. Blue transforms lack of patience and lack of inspiration to health and balance. It calms hyperactivity and helps to communicate better in communication and prayer. Blue helps to: • deal with lack of, patience • deal with lack of faith • deal with hormonal problems • overcome sleep problems **Essential Oils and Incense** Chamomile, Cypress, Geranium, Mint **Herbs and Supplements** Chamomile, Evening Primrose, Iodine, Thyme, Witch Hazel **Food** Raw Fruit, Fish, Asparagus, Blueberries, Black Berries, Plums **Gemstones** Blue Agate, Lapis Lazuli, Sapphire, Sodalite **Affirmation** I allow myself to express freely, I assert myself.	Use **indigo** to restore inspiration, imagination and intellect. Indigo transforms obsessions and fears to insight. It harmonizes your wisdom and skills and revitalizes the mind. It stimulates your brain through the power of ideas. Indigo helps to: • deal with hormonal problems • deal with tension and fear • deal with mental fatigue and other psychological problems • deal with calcium deficiency **Essential Oils and Incense** Camphor, Frankincense, Myrrh, Patchouli, Star Anise **Herbs and Supplements** Melatonin, Passionflower **Food** Broccoli, Eggplant, Currants, Grapes, Purple Onions, Prunes **Gemstones** Quartz Crystal, Tanzanite **Affirmation** I may have my own dreams and aspirations.

Crown – Integration of Body and Soul	Communication, Relationship	Love, Compassion, Wisdom
Use **violet** to restore the connection between the physical, creative, intellectual and spiritual aspects of life. Violet balances physical activity and emotional stability and restores your potential to think and learn. **Violet helps to:** • deal with obsessive behaviors • release fears, psychoses • harmonize emotional states • balance overly active glands • restore metabolic equilibrium **Essential Oils and Incense** Jasmine, Myrrh, Magnolia, Lotus **Herbs and Supplements** Mace, Nutmeg **Food** Broccoli, Eggplant, Kale, Plums, Purple Grapes **Gemstones** Amethyst, Clear Quartz **Affirmation** I allow myself to heal and be healed.	Use **turquoise** to restore the ability to concentrate. Turquoise restores control over your state of mental health and balance. Turquoise helps to express truthfully, it balances physical and psychological aspects on the levels of speech and activity. **Turquoise helps to:** • speak your ideas • share inspiration • stimulate immune system • overcome shock **Essential Oils and Incense** Clary Sage, Cypress, Thyme **Herbs and Supplements** Algae, Uva Ursi, Kelp, Nori **Food** Algae, Dulse, Kelp, Nori **Gemstones** Aquamarine, Turquoise, Tourmaline **Affirmation** I am allowed to speak my truth. I deserve to be heard.	Use **pink** to restore inner peace and sacred space. Pink transforms aggression, frustration, and irritation into healing spiritual energy, it helps to overcome fear of death and resolves envy, anger, depression, grief, and grieving. **Pink helps to:** • deal with irritability, worry, grief • deal with grieving • deceive a stubborn though patterns • uplift, calm and soothe oneself **Essential Oils and Incense** Palma Rosa, Rose, Rosewood. **Herbs and Supplements** Rosehip. **Food** Pink Grapefruit, Pink Salmon. **Gemstones** Moonstone, Opal, Rhodonite, Rose Quartz. **Affirmation** I deserve to be seen as being good and pure.

Figure 4.3 Chakra color reference chart.

Therapeutic Uses of Color Therapy

While color therapy is not recognized as a mainstream medical treatment, many individuals find it beneficial for reducing stress, improving mood, and promoting a sense of balance and harmony. It is important to note that color therapy should not replace conventional medical care but can be used as a complementary practice to support overall well-being. Chromotherapy is also used for anxiety, stress, depression, dementia, traumatic brain injury, infections, fatigue, pain, cramps, headache, migraine headache, diabetes, hypertension, and many other conditions (Hart, 2022).

Evidence-Based Effects of Color Therapy

Color therapy has been used to promote mental health, cognitive abilities, and well-being. One group of researchers studied 135 older adults who were placed in groups where red, green, or white lights were the intervention. They found that green and red light therapies demonstrated a modest improvement in cognitive abilities (Paragas et al., 2019). Others have studied the impact of color therapy on stress, with one group of researchers finding no significant difference between a control group and an experimental group when using virtual color therapy rooms (Vaquero-Blasco et al., 2020). In another study of 150 college students, color therapy using blue chromotized water intake three times a day following meals for 6 weeks and watching blue glass sheets for 15–20 minutes before sleeping for 6 weeks demonstrated, when compared to a control group, a significant improvement in anxiety. These researchers concluded that 453 nm (blue color) was an effective intervention for anxiety in college students (Azemia et al., 2018).

Potential Adverse Effects and Concerns

Color therapy uses colors to promote physical and emotional well-being. While it is considered safe and noninvasive, some individuals may experience certain adverse effects. These effects are usually mild and short-lived. For example, some people may feel overly stimulated or agitated when exposed to bright or intense colors, particularly if they are sensitive to light or have certain neurological conditions. Others may not experience any noticeable effects at all. It is important to note that the effects of color therapy can vary from person to person.

If you are considering color therapy, it is advisable to consult with a trained professional or therapist who can assess your individual needs and guide you through the process. They can help ensure that the therapy is appropriate and safe for you, considering any potential risk factors or contraindications you may have.

Nurse Guidance for Use of Color Therapy

Nurses need to focus on emotional support. Color therapy can have psychological and emotional benefits, such as promoting relaxation, reducing anxiety, and enhancing mood. Nurses can offer emotional support by actively listening to clients, providing empathy, and creating a calming environment that facilitates the therapeutic effects of color.

Depending on the setting and specific interventions, nurses may be directly involved in administering color therapy. This can be involved in using specific-colored lights, coordinating with other departments for access to color therapy rooms, or facilitating any necessary equipment or supplies. At all points, the nurse must educate themselves on the form of color therapy being used and the equipment involved. The patient's response must be evaluated during and post–color therapy. Nurses play a vital role in monitoring clients during color therapy sessions. They observe clients' physical and emotional responses, such as changes in blood pressure, heart rate, or mood. This monitoring helps ensure the therapy's safety and effectiveness while making any necessary adjustments to the intervention.

Nurses document the outcomes of color therapy sessions and evaluate their effectiveness in achieving the desired goals. This documentation aids in tracking progress and sharing information with the health care team, allowing for ongoing adjustments to the overall care plan. It is important to note that while nurses can support and facilitate color therapy, they should always work within their scope of practice and collaborate with other trained professionals in implementing therapeutic interventions.

Types of Special Education Required

There is no standard education or training for therapists using color therapy. Color therapy is not a licensed health practice the United States. To become a color therapist, there are several educational paths you can pursue. While color therapy might not have universally standardized requirements, here are some common educational approaches you can consider:

- **Research and self-study**: Start by gaining a strong theoretical foundation in color therapy. Conduct research, read books, and study various resources on the subject. This will help you understand the principles, techniques, and benefits of color therapy.
- **Certification programs:** Look for reputable certification programs or courses specifically focused on color therapy. These programs are often designed to provide comprehensive knowledge and practical skills in the field. Research different programs to find the one that aligns with your goals.
- **Alternative medicine or holistic health programs:** Consider enrolling in alternative medicine or holistic health programs that include color therapy as part of their curriculum. These programs provide a broader understanding of complementary therapies and allow you to specialize in color therapy.
- **Continuing education:** Even after completing initial education or certification, stay updated on the latest advancements and research in color therapy. Attend workshops, seminars, or webinars conducted by experienced practitioners or organizations in the field.

Remember to check the credibility and accreditation of any institution or program before enrolling. Additionally, gaining practical experience through internships or apprenticeships can enhance your understanding and skills. Building a network within the color therapy community can also be helpful for professional growth and sharing knowledge.

It is important to note that the requirements for becoming a color therapist may vary across different countries or regions. Therefore, it is advisable to research the specific guidelines and regulations in your area to ensure you meet the necessary educational requirements.

Electrotherapy

Electrotherapy includes several interventions that use electricity for therapeutic reasons. These therapies include transcutaneous electrical nerve stimulation (TENS), electrical nerve stimulation, neuromuscular electrical stimulation (NMES), electroacupuncture, electrically charged magnet therapy, iontophoresis, interferential current, and high-voltage galvanic current (Table 4.2). Electrotherapy usually includes a small device powered by batteries, which is connected via wires to adhesive pads, which are placed on the skin. When the unit is turned on, the flow of electrical current is delivered. Usually, a dial controls the amount of electrical current that is delivered. As nurses, we are familiar with defibrillators, which work much in the same way, but of course deliver a much higher voltage of energy to restart the cardiac rhythm. The therapies used do vary in the effects, electrical waveforms, and frequencies (Revord, 2017).

Electrotherapy equipment can range in cost, can be administered only in health centers and clinics by experienced clinicians or those trained in their use, or patients can be taught to manage their electrotherapy in their homes. The FDA is responsible for verifying that devices used are safe and pose no danger to the public (Revord, 2017). The FDA does not determine if the devices are effective. That is the responsibility of clinical researchers. Electrical stimulation should not be delivered over malignancies or areas that are infected or that have broken skin (Revord, 2017).

Table 4.2 Types of Electrotherapies

Transcutaneous electrical neuromuscular stimulation (TENS)	TENS is an application of surface electrodes to deliver mild electrical current using a small battery-operated device called a TENS unit. (Amer-Cuenca et al., 2023).

Table 4.2 Types of Electrotherapies

Neuromuscular electrical stimulation (NMES)	NMES is a treatment that delivers electrical impulses to nerves, which cause the muscles to contract, mimicking natural muscle movement (Physiopedia, 2023).
Percutaneous electrical nerve stimulation (PENS)	Percutaneous nerve stimulation is used by experts in neuromodulation with the aim to stimulate nerves for a natural biological response or to apply pharmaceuticals in tiny doses at the site of action (Physiopedia, 2023).
Iontophoresis	Iontophoresis is a treatment in which low-intensity electric current is passed through the skin, which is soaked in tap water, allowing ionized or charged particles to cross the normal skin barrier, serving as a transdermal drug delivery intervention (Physiopedia, 2023).
Interferential current (IFC)	Refers to the use of two medium frequency alternating currents to yield an amplitude modulated current at 2–250 Hz.
High-voltage galvanic stimulation (HVGC)	Using galvanic stimulation, with direct current modalities that deliver a unidirectional, uninterrupted current without destroying tissue of the patient and within their level of tolerance.
Transcutaneous electrical acustimulation (TEAS)	TEAS is a combination of traditional Chinese acupuncture and TENS (Wang et al., 2014).
Electromagnetic therapy	Low intensity electrical current is applied to acupuncture points with no puncture of the skin (Natural Medicines, 2022).
Electrical stimulation (ES)	ES is a type of PT that involves applying electric current to strengthen muscles, block pain signals, and improve blood circulation

Therapeutic Uses of Electrotherapies

Electrical stimulation (ES) is a type of physical therapy treatment, but it is also used by naturopaths. It involves applying electric current to the muscles. The function of ES is to block pain, strengthen muscles, and improve circulation (Inverarity, 2023). It may be used as a part of rehabilitation. Electrotherapy can be used for many different types of chronic pain tissues such as diabetic nerve pain, fibromyalgia pain, and migraine headaches. It has also been used for would healing and to stimulate bone growth. The mechanism of pain relief with electrotherapy is not entirely clear, but it is theorized that it may block transmission of nociceptive stimuli along nerves or stimulate the release of endorphins, which are natural opiates in the body (Revord, 2017). The types of electric stimulation will be reviewed here. Electrical stimulation has been used to boost attention, memory, and manage neurovascular diseases in the form of transcranial magnetic stimulation for depression and obsessive-compulsive therapy; electroconvulsive therapy for severe depression, and deep brain stimulations to manage the epilepsy or tremors associated with Parkinson's disease. Since this therapy is part of traditional care, we will not discuss it.

Transcutaneous electrical neuromuscular stimulation (TENS) is commonly used for pain management, particularly in chronic pain conditions. It works by stimulating sensory nerves to reduce pain signals reaching the brain. Electrodes are applied to the body over areas that are painful. The intensity of the electricity is adjusted.

Neuromuscular electrical stimulation (NMES), on the other hand, focuses on stimulating muscle contractions to improve muscle strength, prevent atrophy, and aid in rehabilitation (Blazevich et al., 2019). Electroacupuncture combines the principles of acupuncture with electrical stimulation, providing a modality that may enhance pain relief and promote physical healing (Wilson, 2019).

Iontophoresis is used to help provide medication during physical therapy treatments. Medicine is used to decrease both inflammation and muscle spasms. The electric current that is delivered during iontophoresis is used to push medications through your skin and into the body. Medications may also be used to break up calcium deposits that occur, as does in the painful condition of shoulder calcific tendonitis (Inverarity, 2023).

Interferential current (IFC) refers to the use of two medium-frequency alternating currents to yield an amplitude modulated current at 2–250 Hz. IFC involves using four electrodes attached in a crisscross pattern, which causes electrical currents to interfere with one another, permitting the administration of a high-intensity current while still being comfortable for the patient. It is used to improve blood flow to tissues, decrease muscle spasms, and decrease pain (Inverarity, 2023).

High-voltage galvanic stimulation (HVGC) "uses high-voltage and low-frequency electricity to penetrate deep into tissues" (Inverarity, 2023, para. 24). Transcutaneous electrical acustimulation (TEAS) has been shown to be effective for a decline in memory and thinking abilities after surgery, improving bowel function after surgery, prevention of nausea and vomiting after surgery, and improving pain after surgery in some people (Natural Medicines, 2022). The ReliefBand is the most common acustimulation device, is worn on the wrist like how one might wear a watch, and administers an electric current on the wrist. The FDA has approved it. It is advertised as being effective for nausea induced by all sorts of conditions such as anxiety, seasickness, hangovers, morning sickness, and several other causes (ReliefBand, 2023).

Other sources of treatment can be accomplished by applying a TENS unit to acupuncture points. A HANS dual-channel unit can also be used in much the same way. Common acupuncture points used are the P6 Neiguan point on the wrist for nausea and vomiting and the ST36 Zusanli point below the knee, used to manage gastrointestinal discomfort, fatigue, and stress. Sessions usually last for 30–60 minutes, for 2–7 days a week for 2–12 weeks (Natural Medicines, 2022). There is no known interaction with foods, supplements, or medications. This has been demonstrated to be a safe intervention for use, but more research is necessary to conclusively demonstrate its effectiveness.

Electromagnetic therapy is the use of magnets that have an electric charge whereas static magnet therapy is the use of wearable magnets that touch the skin (Ellis, 2023). It could be in the form of wearable bracelet, magnetized jewelry, or a shoe insole. Special mattresses are made with magnets sewn into them. Magnets are also used with acupuncture and are placed in the same sections of the skin that the acupuncturist uses (Ellis, 2023). Most magnet field therapy is used for the treatment of different types of pain. It has been studied for its use for arthritis pain, insomnia, headaches, wound healing, and fibromyalgia pain. It is safe to wear low-intensity magnets, but it may not be a good idea if you have a pacemaker, an insulin pump, or you are pregnant (Ellis, 2023). Magnets should be taken off for an X-ray or when getting an MRI. It is rare to have side effects, but it is possible to develop pain, nausea, and/or dizziness (Ellis, 2023).

With the use of electromagnets, an electric current is passed through a wire coil, which contains magnetic material. Pulsed electromagnetic field therapy (PEMF) is used to relieve pain and improve patients functioning in musculoskeletal pain conditions. These devices have been shown to be safe and have been approved by the FDA. Magnet therapy has been helpful for some with pain, but research findings have been inconclusive (National Center for Complementary and Integrative Therapies, 2023).

Evidence-Based Effects of Electrotherapies

The research on the effectiveness of electrotherapy has been mixed and is dependent on which type of electrotherapy is being used and for which conditions. We will review a small sample of research literature on some types of electrotherapies. The reader is encouraged to do a search of the literature if they have an interest in a particular type of electrotherapy for a particular clinical purpose. We will review a few examples of evidence to demonstrate the great promise some of these therapies have for managing illness and promoting health and wellness.

One group of researchers set out to identify both the efficacy and safety of TEAS for postoperative pain in laparoscopy by completing a systematic review and meta-analysis of randomized control trials. They found that TEAS can relieve pain in the short-term after laparoscopy, reduce the use of analgesics post-op, decrease the length of stay in the hospital, and improve quality of life. No safety concerns were identified in this study (Meng et al., 2022).

Ahmad (2008) reported on the effectiveness of high-voltage galvanic stimulation (HVPC) in an experimental group testing three different lengths of therapy against a sham treatment for wound healing. The wound surface area (WSA) was used to determine outcomes after 3 to 5 weeks of treatment. There was a significant reduction in the WSA in the 60-minute and 120-minute group compared to the 45-minute and control group. It was demonstrated that the HVPC for 60 and 120 minutes 7 days a week was the optimal duration for enhancing chronic dermal ulcer healing (Ahmad, 2008).

In another study, percutaneous versus transcutaneous electrical nerve stimulation for the treatment of musculoskeletal pain was investigated through a systematic review and meta-analysis. Researchers found that overall, the PENS on pain was statistically but not clinically superior to TENS (Beltran-Alacreu et al., 2022). The TENS used does not require a physiotherapist to deliver the treatment and is able to be provided at home, making it a superior treatment.

Several types of electrotherapies are helpful in managing pain, but more research is needed before any definitive conclusions can be made. For now, if a patient is experiencing musculoskeletal pain, it is prudent to try these therapies to see if they are effective. Chronic pain has its own negative effects, and if these can be avoided it is beneficials to clients, their families, and the communities they live in.

Potential Adverse Effects and Concerns

While electrical stimulation therapy can have beneficial effects, it is important to be aware of potential adverse effects. Some possible adverse effects of electrical stimulation therapy include the following:

1. **Skin irritation:** Prolonged or high-intensity electrical stimulation may cause skin irritation at the electrode sites. This can manifest as redness, itching, or a rash. Proper skin preparation and electrode placement can help minimize this risk. Some people with more sensitive skin may be more prone to this. If it happens the treatment should be stopped, and a soothing lotion should be applied to the affected area (Inverarity, 2023). Burns rarely happen but can if the intensity used is too great. Appropriate skin care for burns should be applied, and this can be prescribed by a primary care provider.
2. **Muscle soreness**: Intense electrical stimulation can cause muscle soreness, like what one might experience after an intense workout. This soreness is typically temporary and subsides within a few days.
3. **Muscle spasms:** In some cases, electrical stimulation may induce unintended muscle contractions or spasms. These involuntary contractions can be uncomfortable or even painful. Adjusting the parameters of stimulation or discontinuing the therapy can usually resolve this issue.
4. **Discomfort or pain:** While electrical stimulation is tolerable, some individuals may experience discomfort or pain during the therapy. Adjustments in intensity or frequency can help alleviate these issues, but it is important to communicate any discomfort to the health care provider. Muscle tearing, although rare, is possible. Electrical stimulation should be stopped immediately with intense

muscle pain (Inverarity, 2023).

5. **Interference with implants:** Individuals with pacemakers, defibrillators, or other implanted devices should exercise caution when considering electrical stimulation therapy. It is crucial to consult with the health care provider to ensure that the therapy will not interfere with the functioning of these devices.

These adverse effects are typically mild and temporary. However, it is important to discuss any concerns or potential risks with a qualified health care professional before undergoing electrical stimulation therapy. They can provide personalized guidance based on your specific health conditions and needs.

Nurse Guidance for Use of Electrotherapy

The role of nurses in assisting patients with electrical stimulation therapy is crucial in improving patient outcomes and promoting their well-being. Nurses play a comprehensive role in assessing, planning, implementing, and evaluating the use of electrical stimulation devices for therapeutic purposes. Here are some key aspects of the nurse's role in this process:

1. **Assessment:** Nurses are responsible for conducting a thorough assessment of the patient's condition, including their medical history, current health status, and specific needs. They collaborate with other health care professionals to determine if electrical stimulation is appropriate and safe for the patient. Assessing during the therapy for the level of pain so excess irritation can be avoided is prudent. Also assessing the skin for any irritation or burns post-therapy is essential.
2. **Patient education:** Nurses educate patients about the purpose, benefits, and potential risks associated with electrical stimulation therapy. They provide information about the device, its set-up and proper usage, ensuring that patients understand how to operate and care for the equipment. Patient education empowers individuals to actively participate in their own treatment and promotes adherence to therapy. Further, patients should be taught about the potential adverse effects so that they can be on the lookout for any issues before they become severe. Patients should also be

encouraged to report any skin irritation, burns, or increases in pain to both their therapist and their primary provider so that electrotherapy can be altered and care for the skin can be provided.

3. **Device selection and application:** Nurses collaborate with the health care team to select the appropriate electrical stimulation device for the patient's condition. They ensure proper electrode placement and settings based on the desired therapeutic outcome. Moreover, they monitor and adjust the stimulation parameters as per the patient's response.
4. **Safety and infection control:** Nurses prioritize patient safety by adhering to infection-control measures and ensuring proper hygiene during the use of electrical stimulation devices. They conduct regular inspections of the equipment, maintain cleanliness, and educate patients on infection prevention strategies. Following safety protocols helps minimize the risk of complications. An article by Manana-Kurak et al. (2020) highlights the importance of infection-control practices in electrical stimulation therapy to prevent health care–associated infections.
5. **Evaluation and documentation:** Nurses document the patient's response to electrical stimulation therapy, including any progress or adverse effects. They collaborate with the health care team to evaluate the effectiveness of the treatment and modify the plan if necessary. Accurate documentation ensures continuity of care and facilitates communication among health care professionals.

It is worth noting that the nurse's role in electrical stimulation therapy may vary depending on the specific health care setting, patient population, and scope of practice. Therefore, nurses should follow their institutional guidelines and collaborate with other health care professionals to ensure optimal patient care. Some nurses may deliver the therapy themselves and when they do, need to be especially vigilant about learning how to properly use the device and what special precautions are needed. A search for evidence-based information on the device should be obtained before using it.

Types of Special Education Required

To provide electrical stimulation therapy, health care providers typically require specialized education and training. This education includes a comprehensive understanding of the physiological principles underlying electrical stimulation, knowledge of different electrical stimulation modalities, and expertise in device selection and application. Additionally, health care professionals need to be proficient in assessing patients' conditions and determining the appropriateness of electrical stimulation for their specific needs. To acquire this knowledge and skill set, professionals may pursue specialized courses, workshops, or certification programs focused on electrical stimulation therapy. Continuous learning and staying up-to-date with advancements in the field are essential for providing effective and safe electrical stimulation.

Heat and Cold Therapy

Heat and cold therapies involve the application of temperature to affected areas of the body for therapeutic purposes. Heat therapy, also referred to as thermotherapy, such as the use of heating pads or warm baths, can help alleviate muscle stiffness, increase blood flow, and soothe soreness. It is often used in the management of musculoskeletal conditions like arthritis and back pain.

On the other hand, cold therapy, also known as cryotherapy, involves the application of ice packs or cold compresses to reduce inflammation and relieve pain. Cryotherapy can help numb an area, decrease swelling, and facilitate healing after acute injuries. Both heat and cold therapy have demonstrated benefits in pain management and post-injury recovery. However, it is important to use caution and follow proper guidelines to avoid burns or skin damage.

Throughout time and all around the world people have used both cold and heat therapy for health and wellness. In ancient Greece and Rome, bathing in thermal baths was used, and they believed the waters had healing properties. The tradition of the Finish sauna is still used extensively today and is both cleansing and restorative (Payne, 2023). Thermotherapy and cryotherapy are commonly used in health care for various therapeutic purposes. Let us discuss each of these in more depth.

Therapeutic Uses of Heat Therapy

Heat therapy helps alleviate muscle pain, joint stiffness, and menstrual cramps by increasing blood flow, relaxing muscles, and reducing muscle spasms. Applying heat can promote relaxation, relieve stress, and provide comfort. Heat applications dilate blood vessels, improve blood flow, and in turn accelerate tissue healing. Heat is often utilized in physical therapy to enhance the effectiveness of exercises, increase joint flexibility, and reduce joint contractures. Heat therapy aids in the healing process by promoting tissue repair, reducing inflammation, and relieving pain associated with sprains, strains, and other injuries.

Therapeutic Uses of Cold Therapy

Cold therapy reduces pain by numbing the affected area, reducing nerve activity, and limiting inflammation in conditions such as sprains, strains, and arthritis. Applying cold aids in reducing swelling by constricting blood vessels and limiting the accumulation of fluid.

Cold therapy is frequently used for acute sports injuries like ankle sprains, muscle strains, and bruises to limit swelling, alleviate pain, and accelerate recovery. Applying cold to the head or neck can help alleviate headaches, migraines, and sinus pain by constricting blood vessels and reducing inflammation.

Evidence-Based Effects of Heat and Cold Therapy

Researchers reviewed 104 studies that focused on swimming in cold water. They concluded that swimming in cold water helps to reduce both insulin resistance and fat in men (Payne, 2023). A 2016 study demonstrated that subjects who took cold showers used fewer sick days from work. Payne (2023) reviewed several other results, including lifelong sauna used linked to reduced risk of heart and neurodegenerative disease; heat application in arthritis, menstrual cramps, and lower back pain is helpful; and cold helps with acute injuries, reducing pain, inflammation, and swelling.

In one study on the effects of cooling therapies on those with multiple sclerosis (MS) using a meta-analysis technique, researchers found cooling therapies to have a beneficial effect on fatigue, physical activity, and quality of life in persons with MS (Bilgin et al., 2022).

Hsu et al. (2022) used a systematic review and a meta-analysis to study cold intervention for relieving migraine symptoms and found that cold interventions had a short-term effect on reducing migraine pain compared to noncold regimens but the cold interventions had marginal longer-term effects of relieving migraine pain.

Potential Adverse Effects and Concerns

Heat and cold therapies have various potential adverse effects that should be considered. Heat therapy, such as using heating pads or hot packs, can lead to burns or skin irritation if applied for too long or at excessively high temperatures. Cold therapy, like using ice packs or cold baths, may cause frostbite or skin damage if applied directly to the skin without a barrier. Both therapies can potentially cause numbness or sensation loss if applied for extended periods. It is important to follow recommended usage guidelines, monitor skin condition, and prioritize safety. Always consult with a health care professional for specific advice. When using cold or heat therapy on patients with neuropathic changes such as diabetic patients or older adults, one must use special care to not cause harm as these patients may lack the sensation to recognize when the stimulus is too hot or too cold.

Nurse Guidance for Use of Heat and Cold Therapy

The role of nurses in providing heat or cold therapy is essential in promoting patient comfort and facilitating the therapeutic effects of these treatments. Nurses assess the patient's condition and determine if heat or cold therapy is appropriate based on the health care provider's orders or treatment plan. They educate patients about the benefits, risks, and proper application of heat or cold therapy. Nurses also ensure the safety of patients by monitoring vital signs, skin integrity, and the duration of therapy. They may assist patients in applying or removing heat or cold packs, ensuring the correct temperature, and ensuring proper skin protection. Nurses provide ongoing evaluation, document patient responses, and communicate any adverse effects to the health care team. Special consideration needs to be made for those clients who have decreased sensation such as diabetics and older adults as they may not recognize intense burning or cold sensations from damaging levels of cold or heat.

Types of Special Education Required

To perform cold therapy, sometimes referred to as cryotherapy, the individual providing the treatment would ideally have a background in health care, such as being a licensed health care professional or a certified cryotherapy technician. While specific education requirements may vary depending on the jurisdiction and facility, some common educational components for cryotherapy practitioners include a basic knowledge of human anatomy and physiology; an understanding of cryotherapy principles, techniques, and safety protocols; familiarity with the various cryotherapy modalities and equipment; training in assessing patient suitability for cryotherapy and identifying contraindications; knowledge of potential adverse effects and how to mitigate them; and awareness of emergency procedures and first aid protocols. It is essential to check the local regulations and requirements as they may differ based on location. Training programs, certifications, and continuing education courses can provide the necessary knowledge and skills for safe and effective cryotherapy administration.

In this chapter several select therapies were discussed that impact the body physically, including chiropractic/osteopathic manipulation, massage therapy, light stimulation, electrical stimulation, color therapy, and heat and cold therapy. Although the mechanisms of action of each of these therapies is believed to be physiological, such as creating vasodilation, or vasoconstriction, one cannot deny that these therapies may have psychological benefits also.

Discussion Questions for Your Consideration

1. Please share one therapy from this chapter that you have personally experienced or that you delivered to your patients/clients. Explain the physiological changes that occur in the body and focus on the condition that has been treated. For example, if you used ice on a sprained ankle, how did it work to reduce pain? How effective on a scale from 0–10 was their therapy for the condition treated? What precautions should be used for the physical type of complementary care therapy?
2. Please describe proper education or training in your state for one of the physical therapies presented in this chapter. Do you think the

educational requirements are adequate and provide for the safety of patients and clients?

Experiential Activities

1. Consider participating in massage, color therapy, heat/cold therapy, or any other therapy discussed in this chapter when appropriate. Write up a synopsis of the therapy session addressing the following: benefits of the therapy, effectiveness for the health issue, adverse or unpleasant effects of therapy, and both the knowledge and the preparedness of your therapist. What did you like about the therapy? What did you not like about the therapy?
2. Interview an individual who provides massage, electrical stimulation, color therapy, and heat and cold therapy and ask them to discuss the following:
    a. How did they learn how to provide the therapy? What education and experience did they have before practicing alone?
    b. What positive results have they seen in patients or clients?
    c. Have any of their clients ever reported any adverse effects?
    d. What conditions respond most favorably to the treatment with the therapy?

References

Ahmad, E. T. (2008). High voltage pulsed galvanic stimulation: Effect of treatment duration on healing of chronic pressure ulcers. *Annals of Burns and Fire Disasters*, *21*(3), 124–128.

Amer-Cuenca, J. J., Badenes-Ribera, L., Biviá-Roig, G., Arguisuelas, M. D., Suso, M. L., & Lisón, J. F. (2023). The dose-dependent effects of transcutaneous electrical nerve stimulation for pain relief in individuals with fibromyalgia: A systematic review and meta-analysis. *PAIN*, *164*(8), 1645–1657. https://doi.org/10.1097/j.pain.0000000000002876

Angelopoulou, E., Anagnostouli, M., Chrousos, G. P., & Bougea, A. (2020). Massage therapy as a complementary treatment for Parkinson's disease: A systematic literature review. *Complementary Therapies in Medicine*, *49*. https://doi.org/10.1016/j.ctim.2020.102340

Azeemi, S., Iram, H., Younas, Q., & Azeem, A. (2018) Effect of blue colour (453 nm visible range radiation) on anxiety in college students. Chinese Medicine, 9, 1–6. https://doi.org/10.4236/cm.2018.91001

Beltran-Alacreu, H., Serrano-Muñoz, D., Álvarez, D. M.-C., Fernández-Pérez, J. J., Gómez-Soriano, J., & Avendaño-Coy, J. (2022). Percutaneous versus transcutaneous electrical nerve stimulation for the treatment of musculoskeletal pain: A systematic review and meta-analysis. *Pain Medicine*, *23*(8), 1387–1400. https://doi.org/10.1093/pm/pnac027

Bigos, S. J. (1994). Acute low back problems in adults: Clinical practice guidelines (No. 14). U.S. Department of Health and Human Services.

Bilgin, A., Kesik, G. & Ozdemir, L. (2022). The effects of cooling therapies on fatigue, physical activity, and quality of life in multiple sclerosis. Rehabilitation Nursing, 47(6), 228–236. https://doi.org/10.1097/RNJ.0000000000000388

Blake, E. (2008). Electrotherapy modalities. In L. Chaitow (Ed.), *Naturopathic physical medicine (pp. 539–562).* Churchill Livingstone. https://doi.org/10.1016/B978-044310390-2.50017-1

Blazevich, A. J., Collins, D. F., Millet, G. Y., Vaz, M. A., & Maffiuletti, N. A. (2021). Enhancing adaptations to neuromuscular electrical stimulation training interventions. *Exercise and Sport Sciences Reviews*, *49*(4), 244–252. https://doi.org/10.1249/JES.0000000000000264

Brouwer, A., Nguyen, H. T., Snoek, F. J., van Raalte, D. H., Beekman, A. T. F., Moll, A. C., & Bremmer, M. A. (2017). Light therapy: Is it safe for the eyes? Acta Psychiatrica Scandinavica , 136(6), 534–548. https://doi.org/10.1111/acps.12785

Chang, C. H., Liu, C. Y., Chen, S. J., & Tsai, H. C. (2018) Efficacy of light therapy on nonseasonal depression among elderly adults: A systematic review and meta-analysis. *Neuropsychiatric Disease and Treatment*, 2018, 3091–3102. https://doi.org/10.2147/NDT.S180321

Cheng, K., Martin, L. F., Calligaro, H., Patwardhan, A., & Ibrahim, M. M. (2022). Case report: Green light exposure relieves chronic headache pain in a colorblind patient. Clinical Medicine Insights: Case Reports, 15, 1–7. https://doi.org/10.1177/11795476221125164

Cleveland Clinic. (2023, June 23). *Chiropractic adjustment.* https://my.clevelandclinic.org/health/treatments/21033-chiropractic-adjustment

Coulter, I., Adams, A., Coggan, P. et al. (1998). A comparative study of chiropractic and medical education. *Alternative Therapies in Health and Medicine.*, 4, 64–75.

Cutshall, S. M., Wentworth, L. J., Engen, D., Sundt, T. M , Kelly, R. F., & Bauer, B. A. (2010). Effect of massage therapy on pain, anxiety, and tension in cardiac surgical patients: A pilot study. Complementary Therapies in Clinical Practice, 16, 92–95.

Daily Nurse. (2023, July). *Bedside insight: Amazing nurse discoveries.* https://dailynurse.com/bedside-insight-amazing-nurse-discoveries/

Delaney, J. P. A., Leong, K. S., Watkins, A., & Brodie, D. (2002). The short-term effects of myofascial trigger point massage therapy on cardiac autonomic tone in healthy subjects. Journal of Advanced Nursing, 37, 364–371.

Diego, M. A., & Field, T. (2009). Moderate pressure massage elicits a parasympathetic nervous system. response. The International Journal of Neuroscience, 119, 630–638.

Ellis, R. R. (2023, July). What is magnet therapy? WebMD. https://www.webmd.com/pain-management/magnetic-field-therapy-overview

Fang, C.-S., Chang, S.-L., Fang, C.-J., & Chou, F.-H. (2023). Effect of massage therapy on sleep quality in critically ill patients: A systematic review and meta-analysis. *Journal of Clinical Nursing*, 32, 4362– 4373. https://doi.org/10.1111/jocn.16660

Funabashi, M., Pohlman, K. A., Goldsworthy, R., Lee, A., Tibbles, A., Mior, S., & Kawchuk, G. (2020). Beliefs, perceptions and practices of chiropractors and patients about mitigation strategies for benign adverse events after spinal manipulation therapy. *Chiropractic & Manual Therapies*, *28*(1). https://doi.org/10.1186/s12998-020-00336-3

Gupta, R. (2021, February). Color therapy in mental health and wellbeing. International Journal of All Research Education and Scientific Methods, 9(2), 1068–1076.

Hart, J. (2022). Chromotherapy: Color and light therapies may benefit health. Integrative & Complementary Therapies, 28(2), 104–106. https://doi.org/10.1089/ict.2022.29012.jha

Horn, D., Ehret, D., Suresh, G., & Soll, R. (2019). Sunlight for the prevention and treatment of hyperbilirubinemia in term and late preterm neonates. *The Cochrane Database of Systematic Reviews, 2019*(3). https://doi.org/10.1002/14651858.CD013277

Hsu, Y., Chen, C., Wu, S., & Chen, K. (2023). Cold intervention for relieving migraine symptoms: A systematic review and meta-analysis. Journal of Clinical Nursing, 32(11/12), 2455–2465. https://doi.org/10.1111/jocn.16368

Inverarity, L. (2023, July). How electrical stimulation is used in physical therapy. VeryWellHealth. https://www.verywellhealth.com/electrical-stimulation-2696122

Jagan, S., Park, T., & Papathanassoglou, E. (2019), Effects of massage on outcomes of adult intensive care unit patients: a systematic review. Nursing and Critical Care, 24, 414–429. https://doi.org/10.1111/nicc.12417

Leonard, J. (2020, April). LED light therapy for skin: Does it work? Medical News Today. https://www.medicalnewstoday.com/articles/led-light-therapy

Lowe, W. (2023, April 1). Massage in pain management. *Massage Magazine*, (323), p. 20.

Manana-Kurak, G., Fazekas, B., Tsoncheva, M., et al. (2020). Infection control and work safety compliance in the operating room: A self-report survey of nurses in eastern Hungary. The American Journal of Infection Control, 48(10).

Meng, D., Mao, Y., Song, Q., Yan, C., Zhao, Q., Yang, M., Xiang, G., & Song, Y. (2022). Efficacy and safety of transcutaneous electrical acupoint stimulation (TEAS) for postoperative pain in laparoscopy: A systematic review and meta-analysis of randomized controlled trials. *Evidence-Based Complementary & Alternative Medicine (ECAM)*, 1–17. https://doi.org/10.1155/2022/9922879

Miri, S., Hosseini, S. J., Ghorbani Vajargah, P., Firooz, M., Takasi, P., Mollaei, A., Ramezani, S., Tolouei, M., Emami Zeydi, A., Osuji, J., Farzan, R., & Karkhah, S. (2023). Effects of massage therapy on pain and anxiety intensity in patients with burns: A systematic review and meta-analysis. International Wound Journal, 20(6), 2440–2458. https://doi.org/10.1111/iwj.14089

Mollà-Casanova, S., Sempere-Rubio, N., Muñoz-Gómez, E., Aguilar-Rodríguez, M., Serra-Añó, P., & Inglés, M. (2023). Effects of massage therapy alone or together with passive mobilizations on weight gain and length of hospitalization in preterm infants: Systematic review and meta-analysis. Early Human Development, 182. https://doi.org/10.1016/j.earlhumdev.2023.105790

Moyer, C. A. (2011, January 1). Does massage therapy reduce cortisol? A comprehensive quantitative review. *Journal of Bodywork and Movement Therapies*, 15(1), 3-14. doi: 10.1016/j.jbmt.2010.06.001. Epub 2010 Jul 2. PMID: 21147413.

National Center for Complementary and Integrative Health (2023a, June). *Chiropractic in Depth: Education and Licensure of Practitioners.* https://www.nccih.nih.gov/health/chiropractic-in-depth

National Center for Complementary and Integrative Health (2023b, July). Magnets for pain: What you need to know. https://www.nccih.nih.gov/health/magnets-for-pain-what-you-need-to-know

National Center for Complementary and Integrative Health. (2023c, June). Massage therapy: What you need to know. https://www.nccih.nih.gov/health/massage-therapy-what-you-need-to-know

Natural Medicines. (2020, November). Color therapy. [monograph]. http://natural medicines.therapeutic research.com.

Natural Medicines. (2022, March). Electrical acustimulation. [monograph]. http://natural medicines.therapeutic research.com.

Natural Medicines. (2023, March). Light therapy. [monograph]. http://natural medicines.therapeutic research.com.

Paragas, E. D, Ng, A. T. Y., Reyes, D. V. L., et al. Effects of chemotherapy on the cognitive ability of older adults: A quasi-experimental study. *Explore, 15,* 191–197.

Payne, L. (2023). At-home hot and cold therapy: Enjoy the many restorative benefits. Alive: Canada's Natural Health & Wellness Magazine, 487, pp. 39–43.

Physiopedia. (2023a, July). Iontophoresis. https://www.physio-pedia.com/

Iontophoresis?utm_source=physiopedia&utm_medium=search&utm_campaign=ongoing_internal
Physiopedia. (July 2023b). Neuromuscular and muscular electrical stimulation (NMES). https://www.physio-pedia.com/Neuromuscular_and_Muscular_Electrical_Stimulation_(NMES)
Physiopedia. (July 2023c). Percutaneous nerve stimulation. https://www.physio-pedia.com/Percutaneous_Electrical_Nerve_Stimulation?utm_source=physiopedia&utm_medium=search&utm_campaign=ongoing_internal
ReliefBand. (July, 2023). https://www.reliefband.com/?gclid=CjwKCAjwzo2mBhAUEiwAf7wjkoR2A3a366dqDuXwltGfXCSct-bVUlyIluspvXjd-wALSmMjtJEriRoC668QAvD_BwE
Revord, J. (2017b, April 21). How electrotherapy works to ease pain. Spine-Health. https://www.spine-health.com/treatment/pain-management/how-electrotherapy-works-ease-pain
Revord, J. (2017a, April 21). All about electrotherapy and pain relief. Spine-Health. https://www.spine-health.com/treatment/pain-management/all-about-electrotherapy-and-pain-relief#:~:text=Electrotherapy%20includes%20a%20range%20of,to%20improvements%20in%20physical%20functioning
Roseman-Halsband, J. L. (2018). Is color and light therapy an effective complementary therapy for oncology patients? An analysis of one practitioner's anecdotal experiences. *Alternative and Complementary Therapies, 24,* 121–128.
Salehi, A., Hashemi, N., Imanieh, M. H., & Saber, M. (2015). Chiropractic: Is it efficient in treatment of diseases? Review of systematic reviews. *International Journal of Community-Based Nursing and Midwifery*, *3*(4), 244–254.
Terman, M., Terman, J. S., Quitkin, F. M., McGrath, P. J., Stewart, J. W., & Rafferty, B. (1989). Light therapy for seasonal affective disorder: A review of efficacy. *Neuropsychopharmacology, 2*(1), 1–23.
Vahedian-Azimi, A., Ebadi A., Jafarabadi M.A., Saadat, S, & Ahmadi F. (2014). Effect of massage therapy on vital signs and GCS scores of ICU patients: A randomized controlled clinical trial. Trauma Monthly, 19, 1–7.
Vasquero-Blasco, M. A., Perez-Valero, E., Lopez Gordo, M. A., et al. (2020). Virtual reality as a portable alternative to chromotherapy rooms for stress relief: A preliminary study. *Sensors, 20,* 6211.
Vickers, A., & Zollman, C. (1999, October). The manipulative therapies: Osteopathy and chiropractic. British Medical Journal, 319, 1176. https://doi.org/10.1136/bmj.319.7218.1176
Wang, H., Xie, Y., Zhang, Q., Xu, N., Zhong, H., Dong, H., et al. (2014). Transcutaneous electric acupoint stimulation reduces intra-operative remifentanil consumption and alleviates postoperative side-effects in patients undergoing sinusotomy: A prospective, randomized, placebo-controlled trial. *British Journal of Anaesthesia.,* 112, 1075–1082. https://doi.org/10.1093/bja/aeu001
Wilson, D. (2019). Try this: Electroacupuncture. Healthline. https://www.healthline.com/health/electroacupuncture

Credits

Fig. 4.1: Copyright © by Skin58 (CC BY-SA 4.0) at https://commons.wikimedia.org/wiki/File:Blue_Light_acne_phototherapy_iClear.jpg.
Fig. 4.2: Source: https://commons.wikimedia.org/wiki/File:Children_recieving_sun_treatment,_Vienna_Wellcome_L0023936.jpg, 1922.
Fig. 4.3: Adapted from William Vroman, https://commons.wikimedia.org/wiki/File:Chakra_Colors_Reference_Chart.JPG, 2005.

CHAPTER 5

Psychological Therapies

> "A calm mind brings inner strength and self-confidence, so that's very important for good health."
>
> —DALAI LAMA

Objectives

This chapter will enable the reader to do the following:

1. Identify select psychological therapies that are used to promote optimum health and care for common health disorders.
2. Discuss the theoretical rationale for the mode of action of various psychological therapies.
3. Compare and contrast various psychological therapies, including mindfulness, meditation, guided imagery, progressive muscle relaxation, breath work, art therapy, music therapy, dance therapy, and hypnotherapy,
4. Discuss common uses for various psychological therapies in people.
5. Describe evidence-based effects of various psychological therapies.
6. Discuss potential adverse effects to psychological therapies in people.
7. Describe the role of health care providers in guiding patients regarding their use of various psychological therapies.
8. Discuss the role of health care professionals, types of specialized education required, and guidelines for those who wish to help people with using psychological therapies.

Key Terms

Mindfulness: Originating from Buddhist meditation practices, emphasizes the cultivation of nonjudgmental awareness of present-moment experiences.

Meditation: Encompasses a range of practices that promote mental calmness and the ability to focus attention.

Guided imagery: Involves the use of verbal guidance to facilitate visualization, employing all senses to create a multisensory experience.

Progressive muscle relaxation: Involves systematically tensing and relaxing different muscle groups in the body to achieve deep relaxation.

Breath work: The conscious regulation of breathing patterns.

Hypnotherapy: "The use of hypnosis for therapeutic purposes" (Natural Medicines, 2023a, para 1).

Hypnosis: "A state of consciousness with a reduced peripheral awareness and an increased capacity for response to suggestion or instruction" (Natural Medicines, 2023a, para 1).

Art therapy: Allows individuals to express emotions and explore their inner world through various artistic mediums.

Music therapy: Employs the therapeutic use of music, focusing on physical, emotional, cognitive, and social rehabilitation.

Dance/movement therapy (DMT): Defined by the American Dance Therapy Association (ADTA) as the psychotherapeutic use of movement to promote emotional, social, cognitive, and physical integration of the individual.

Introduction

Psychological therapies have become essential tools in the field of mental health, providing individuals with effective ways to manage and overcome various challenges. There has been a significant rise in the utilization of complementary therapies to enhance overall well-being. We will explore and discuss several psychological therapies used as complementary approaches, including mindfulness, meditation, guided imagery, progressive muscle relaxation, breath work, relaxation techniques, hypnotherapy, art therapy, music therapy, and dance therapy. We will delve into their theoretical frameworks, techniques, and benefits.

Stress and Its Negative Impact on Holistic Wellness

Stress is a "state manifested by symptoms that arise from the coordinated activation of the neuroendocrine and immunes systems" (Norris, 2020, p. 128). Hans Selye, renowned endocrinologist, discussed the stress response using his theory general adaptation syndrome to explain stress as an adaptive response involving the entire body as a system that is used to adapt to stressors in one's environment. The stress response involves several clinical manifestations that develop in response to a stressor. The sympathetic nervous system is activated, and this leads to anxiety-related symptoms (Table 5.1).

Theorist, Herbert Benson, 1989, coined the term *relaxation response* and focused on meditative techniques to bring about a response that is opposite to the fight-or-flight responses as seen in the general adaptation syndrome. He explained that just as people can enter the stress response, they can also choose to reverse it, or even prevent it from ever occurring by using relaxation techniques. Benson (1984) recommended techniques, including the use of a mantra to maintain one's focus, deep breathing, and others. He stated that with regular practice of these techniques one would find themselves capable of combatting the stress response with all its negative effects on body and mind. Benson explained that in using these techniques the parasympathetic system could be activated, leading to increased peripheral blood flow, improved activity of natural killer cells, and the production of slow alpha waves in the brain. Also activated is decreased respiratory rate, heart rate, blood pressure, oxygen consumption, muscle tension, epinephrine level, and gastric acidity and motility (Dossey & Keegan, 2022). Why is this so important? There are negative effects of stress in the long-term on the body, and these include problems such as overeating or undereating, anxiety, heart disease, high blood pressure, thoracic angina, headaches, muscle strain, decreased libido, sleep problems, and stomach discomfort (Dossey & Keegan, 2022: Mayo Clinic, 2021; Norris, 2020).

By learning some of the psychological interventions discussed in this chapter people can be taught to manage nagging or even dangerous disorders that threaten their health. Many of these therapies fit nicely in the holistic model of care, which is a patient-centered approach that considers the whole person, including physical, emotional, social, and spiritual aspects of health. This model emphasizes the importance of addressing all aspects of a patient's well-being to promote healing and optimize health outcomes. This is very congruent with psychologically oriented therapies as use of these therapies is believed to be beneficial in interrupting the stress response.

These therapies also help people to be spiritually healthy and help people tap into subconscious feelings and realizations that otherwise would never rise to conscious awareness. Once one becomes conscious of thoughts and feelings that were once buried, they are better able to make connections between thoughts, feelings, and actions and then in turn address issues that were once hidden, often for many years of their life. Many of these therapies are combined with Gestalt therapy sessions to help patients work through their past traumas and psychological challenges.

Most of these psychological therapies are justified by the holistic model of care, discussed in Chapter 2. As a reminder, the holistic model of care is a patient-centered approach that considers the whole person, including physical, emotional, social, and spiritual aspects of health. This model emphasizes the importance of addressing all aspects of a patient's well-being to promote healing and optimize health outcomes. This approach emphasizes the importance of balance and harmony among these several aspects of an individual's life. Holistic care is a health care approach that aims to treat the whole person rather than just the symptoms of a particular illness or condition. Based on this theory and the mind-body-spirit theory, one cannot separate the mind from the body or the body from the mind. We are holistic beings, and there is no real separation of the various parts of us.

Mindfulness

Mindfulness-based interventions, originating from Buddhist meditation practices, emphasize the cultivation of nonjudgmental awareness of present-moment experiences. These techniques have gained significant attention in recent years due to their positive impact on psychological well-being. Research suggests that mindfulness interventions can reduce symptoms of anxiety, depression, and stress (Creswell, 2017).

Table 5.1 Clinical Manifestations of Stress

Psychological Clinical Manifestations	Physiological Clinical Manifestations
Anger Feeling defeated Uneasiness Unhappiness Loss of motivations and concentration Anxiety	Muscular contraction Constricted blood flow to periphery Increase in blood pressure, heart rate, and respiratory rate Difficulty breathing Increase oxygen consumption Shallow breathing Chest constriction

Sources: Dossey and Keegan (2022), Mayo Clinic (2021), Norris (2020).

Participants are encouraged to pay attention to sensations, emotions, and thoughts without any form of judgment.

Therapeutic Uses of Mindfulness

Mindfulness refers to the practice of being fully present and aware of the current moment. It has gained popularity due to its numerous benefits for mental and physical well-being. Mindfulness is used in various contexts, such as stress reduction, anxiety, and depression management, improving focus and attention, enhancing emotional regulation, and promoting overall happiness. Research studies (Hofmann et al., 2010; Khoury et al., 2013) have highlighted the positive effects of mindfulness training. It has been integrated into therapeutic interventions, workplaces, schools, and even health care settings. By cultivating mindfulness, individuals can develop a greater sense of self-awareness, resilience, and inner peace.

Evidence-Based Effects of Mindfulness

One of the primary benefits of mindfulness is stress reduction. Studies have shown that mindfulness-based interventions can effectively reduce perceived stress and physiological markers of stress, such as cortisol levels (Creswell et al., 2014). It can also enhance cognitive flexibility and decrease rumination, which can contribute to lowering anxiety and depression symptoms (Hölzel et al., 2011).

Mindfulness practices have been shown to improve attention and working memory. Regular meditation can enhance both sustained and selective attention, helping individuals focus better and resist distractions (Jha et al., 2007). Furthermore, mindfulness-based interventions have been linked to increased working memory capacity, which is crucial for cognitive functioning (Mrazek et al., 2013).

One group of researchers found, in an experimental study, brief training in mindfulness meditation or somatic relaxation reduces distress and improves positive mood states (Jain et al., 2007). However, "mindfulness meditation may be specific in its ability to reduce distractive and ruminative thoughts and behaviors, and this ability may provide a unique mechanism by which mindfulness meditation reduces distress" (Jain et al., 2007, abstract). Mindfulness practices also, have positive effects on the brain and immune system functioning, potentially enhancing the brain and improving the immune response (Davidson et al., 2003).

In summary, mindfulness practices have demonstrated positive effects on stress reduction, attention, and working memory, as well as physical health outcomes. Incorporating mindfulness into one's daily routine can promote overall well-being and quality of life.

Potential Adverse Effects and Concerns

While mindfulness practices are regarded as beneficial, there are potential adverse effects that can occur. Some individuals may experience symptoms like anxiety, depression, or dissociation when practicing mindfulness. Mindfulness might also exacerbate existing psychological conditions for some individuals. It is crucial to consider these risks, particularly for individuals with a history of trauma or mental health issues. Additionally, studies suggest that poorly trained instructors or improper implementation of mindfulness practices can lead to negative outcomes.

Nurse Guidance for Use of Mindfulness

To guide patients in using mindfulness, nurses can educate patients about the benefits and potential risks of mindfulness. Assessment of patients' readiness and suitability for mindfulness practice needs to occur prior to, during, and after mindfulness practices.

Nurses should also provide guidance on starting with basic mindfulness exercises and gradually progressing to more advanced techniques. Nurses should encourage patients to practice under the guidance of qualified instructors consulting science-based sites such as the the American Holistic Nurses Association, the National Center for Complementary and Integrative Health, and other professionally oriented resources. Nurses can help patients to integrate mindfulness into their daily routines and establish a consistent practice.

Types of Special Education Required

To educate individuals about mindfulness, professionals need appropriate training and expertise. The education required involves gaining knowledge of mindfulness principles, practices, and their psychological and physiological effects. Training programs should cover topics such as the history of mindfulness, different mindfulness techniques, the science behind its benefits, and potential risks. Additionally, understanding cultural, social, and ethical considerations is essential. Education can be obtained through formal programs, workshops, or certifications provided by recognized mindfulness organizations or universities. Professionals can reference resources like books, research articles, and online platforms to stay updated with current information.

Meditation

Meditation, like mindfulness, encompasses a range of practices that promote mental calmness and the ability to focus attention. Techniques such as mindfulness meditation, loving-kindness meditation, and transcendental meditation have been scientifically shown to reduce stress, improve attention, enhance emotional regulation, and increase self-awareness (Tang et al., 2015).

Therapeutic Uses of Meditation

Meditation has a myriad of uses, promoting mental, emotional, and physical well-being. It helps reduce stress, anxiety, and depression, cultivating a sense of calm and clarity. Through focus and awareness, meditation enhances concentration and cognitive abilities. It fosters self-awareness, allowing individuals to understand their thoughts and emotions better. Meditation can aid in managing pain, improving sleep quality, and boosting the immune system. It also enhances empathy and compassion and promotes self-compassion. Furthermore, meditation can deepen spiritual experiences, expand consciousness, and cultivate a sense of inner peace and happiness. It serves as a powerful tool for personal growth and overall holistic well-being.

However, according to the National Center for Complementary and Integrative Health, much of the research on meditation "has been preliminary or not scientifically rigorous. Because the studies examined many diverse types of meditation and mindfulness practices, and the effects of those practices are hard to measure, results from the studies have been difficult to analyze and may have been interpreted too optimistically" (NCCIH, 2023, para. 7).

Evidence-Based Effects of Meditation

Meditation is a practice that has gained immense popularity in recent years due to its potential positive effects on mental and physical well-being. In examining the evidence, one can see effects on body, mind, and spirit. According to a 2017 U.S. survey, the NCCIH (2023) found that adults who practiced meditation over 12 months tripled between 2012 and 2017, from 4.1% to 14.2%. The effects of meditation are difficult to measure in scientific research. The reasons for this dramatic increase in meditation use is because that real people are realizing from this complementary and integrative therapy.

Numerous scientific studies have demonstrated the positive impact of meditation on various aspects of human health. One study by Tang et al. (2007) found that mindfulness meditation can enhance attentional control and cognitive performance. The researchers conducted a randomized controlled trial in which participants who underwent an 8-week meditation training program showed improvement in attention, working memory, and decision-making compared to those in a control group. A meta-analysis by Pascoe et al. (2017) explored the effects of meditation on blood pressure. The study found that regular meditation practice can significantly reduce both systolic and diastolic blood pressure, suggesting its potential role in managing hypertension.

Another study conducted by Goyal et al. (2014) reviewed 47 randomized controlled trials and concluded that meditation has moderate evidence of improving symptoms of anxiety, depression, and pain. Additionally, meditation was found to reduce stress and improve overall psychological well-being.

Potential Adverse Effects and Concerns

Meditation is a safe practice; however, some individuals who have led an incredibly stressful life, and who are quite acclimated to being in an agitated state as a part of their normal existence, may become disturbed initially upon feeling relaxed for the first time in many years. For example, Kuijpers et al. (2007) found that intensive meditation retreats may lead to negative side effects in vulnerable individuals, including increased anxiety and cognitive difficulties. It is crucial to consider individual differences and carefully assess the suitability of specific meditation techniques for different populations.

While meditation offers numerous benefits, it is crucial to recognize that some individuals, particularly those vulnerable to mental health concerns, may experience adverse effects. Supervision, adequate training, and tailored approaches become essential to ensure the safe practice of meditation.

Nurse Guidance for Use of Meditation

The role of the nurse in guiding patients who want to use meditation is to provide support, education, and guidance throughout the process. Nurses can inform patients about the benefits of meditation, its techniques, and how it can complement their existing health care regimen. They can help patients integrate meditation into their daily routines by establishing realistic goals, providing instructions on proper technique, and recommending resources such as meditation apps or classes. Additionally, nurses can offer emotional support, address any concerns or obstacles, and monitor the patient's progress to ensure they are achieving the desired outcomes. Overall, nurses play a crucial role in empowering patients to incorporate meditation as a self-care practice for their overall well-being.

Types of Special Education Required

To become a meditation teacher, various educational routes exist. Formal training programs, such as certification courses offered by recognized meditation organizations, can provide comprehensive instruction in theory and practice. These programs often cover meditation techniques, mindfulness principles, teaching methodologies, and ethical considerations.

Guided Imagery

Guided imagery involves the use of verbal guidance to facilitate visualization, employing all senses to create a multisensory experience. These techniques activate the imagination and enhance relaxation, often guided by a therapist or an audio recording. Guided imagery has shown promise in reducing pain, anxiety, and distress, particularly in cancer patients undergoing treatment. Guided imagery is used to enhance relaxation and at other times to visualize solutions to problems or disease-fighting processes (Natural Medicines, 2022a).

Some researchers have suggested that guided imagery events are experienced as actual events (Kealy & Arbuthnott, 2003). This may be related to the fact that guided imagery with all its sensory and experiential details are like actual places and events and to the finding that visual perception and visual mental imagery are similarly processed (Borst & Kosslyn, 2008).

The guided imagery process can be led by an instructor, or prerecorded tapes can be used. Relaxation therapies or biofeedback can also be integrated with guided imagery to increase therapeutic effects (Natural Medicines, 2022a). The usual prescription for guided imagery is two sessions for 5–15 minutes used daily and often completed upon waking up in the morning and before going to bed at night (Fish, 2018). While using this complementary therapy the individual should find a quiet place and sit up straight, with legs and arms open and unfolded. It helps to maintain closed eyes and to maintain a relaxed posture with face, shoulders, arms, and legs relaxed. Normally the individual takes some deep breaths in and out when they begin an imagery session. A conscious effort should be maintained to use this time to let go of all tension before beginning. Thinking of a safe and peaceful place is helpful (Dossey & Keegan, 2022)

Imagery can improve quality of life by positively impacting one's mood and decreasing stress, which leads to an improvement in health (Dossey & Keegan, 2022). One writer suggested that guided visual imagery can be used for relaxation when faced with stressful experiences (Fish, 2018). This can benefit nurses as well, who can take a small break from their practice by imagining a natural scene, object, or event that allows them to withdraw from outside stimuli for a brief period and once again achieve a relaxed state (Stiller, 2022). It could also impact patients who are at times facing the most stressful circumstances ever encountered in their life.

Therapeutic Uses of Guided Imagery

There are a wide range of uses for guided imagery in different contexts:

- Stress reduction and relaxation: Guided imagery is commonly used to induce relaxation and reduce stress. Through visualization, individuals can imagine serene environments, calming scenes, or pleasant experiences, helping them achieve a state of deep relaxation.
- Pain management: By guiding the mind into vividly imagining pain-free states or distracting from discomfort, guided imagery

has shown promise in alleviating pain. It can be used as a complementary technique alongside medical treatment.

- Performance enhancement: Athletes, musicians, and individuals in various performance-oriented fields use guided imagery to improve focus, confidence, and skill. By vividly imagining successful outcomes and practicing mental rehearsal, individuals can enhance their performance abilities.
- Promoting emotional healing: Guided imagery can assist in emotional healing and psychotherapy by helping individuals process unresolved emotions and traumatic experiences. Visualization techniques can aid in creating new emotional patterns and promoting self-compassion.

Evidence-Based Effects of Guided Imagery

Guided imagery is a widely used complementary therapy that harnesses the power of imagination to promote relaxation, reduce stress, and enhance overall well-being. The evidence-based support for guided imagery among people is promising and shows some benefits for improved physical and mental health.

One source list guided imagery as being "possibly effective" for both postoperative pain and stressful medical situations (Natural Medicines, 2022a). In one randomized control study on the effect of guided imagery on postoperative pain management in 60 patients undergoing lower extremity surgery, researchers found that the differences between a control group and an experimental group receiving guided visual imagery were statistically significant in the short-term postoperative period (Aydin & Dogan, 2023). Researchers mentioned that the findings of their study were like others that studied the impact of guided imagery on postoperative pain (Antall & Kresevic, 2004; Baird et al., 2010). In a study of the impact of guided imagery on fibromyalgia pain, a chronic pain syndrome, it was demonstrated that functional status and feelings of self-efficacy improved, but pain did not (Menzies et al., 2006).

In terms of mental health, guided imagery has shown promise as an adjunctive therapy for individuals with anxiety and depression. A study by Kavitha and Sasikala (2019) found that in 3 months of intervention, guided imagery significantly impacted the quality of life in one sample of individuals with hypertension. Teaching guided imagery and relaxation techniques to nursing students showed positive results, with students indicating that that they benefited from learning the techniques for relaxation, which included guided imagery, and they intended to use them in the future (Windle et al., 2021).

Potential Adverse Effects and Concerns

The potential adverse effects of guided imagery are minimal and rare, making it a safe therapeutic intervention. However, it is important to consider individual variations and potential risks. Few studies have reported adverse effects, but they include rare occurrences such as vivid imagery leading to mild distress or exacerbation of symptoms. A study by Kazdin and Whitley (2019) highlighted the importance of considering contraindications and ensuring appropriate training and supervision while using guided imagery to minimize any potential risks. Many studies using different populations of people have found that guided imagery impacts anxiety. It has been extremely helpful with anxiety management in nursing students, (Speck 1990), patients coping with medical-related anxiety (Serra et al., 2012), and in new mothers (Rees, 1995).

Nurse Guidance for Use of Guided Imagery

When utilizing guided imagery as a complementary therapy for individuals, nurses should consider a few key factors. First, they must conduct an initial assessment to determine the person's comfort level, preferences, and ability to engage in visualization. Nurses should provide a peaceful environment and guide the person through a detailed imagery script, tailored to their specific needs. One must consider if the guided script contains any information in it that could be distressing to patients. For example, it would not be beneficial to guide the patient through a scenario involving the ocean if they once had a near-death drowning incident. This would not have a relaxing effect and in fact could induce trauma. It is crucial to ensure cultural sensitivity and respect personal beliefs and experiences. Additionally, monitoring the person's response during and after the session is essential. By considering these nursing considerations, the potential benefits of guided imagery on individuals' well-being can be maximized.

Types of Special Education Required

To effectively lead people through guided imagery, it is essential for health care professionals to have a solid educational foundation. Recommended education may include graduate programs or workshops in psychology, counseling, or integrative medicine. Courses focusing on mindfulness, visualization techniques, and therapeutic communication would also be beneficial. It would be beneficial to consult with professional organizations such as the American Holistic Nurses Association to obtain programs on guided imagery preparation that they endorse. Now we will discuss another technique for relaxation called progressive muscle relaxation.

Progressive Muscle Relaxation

Progressive muscle relaxation (PMR) involves systematically tensing and relaxing different muscle groups in the body to achieve deep relaxation. By practicing PMR, individuals develop greater body awareness and reduced muscle tension and experience overall relaxation. PMR was developed by Dr. Edmund Jacobson 50 years ago (Bourne, 2005). Dr. Jacobson discovered that a muscle could effectively be relaxed by first tensing it up for a few seconds and then releasing it. He also discovered that one could do this through the whole body and achieve a deep state of relaxation. PMR works best for people who have anxiety that is associated with muscular tension (Bourne, 2005). PMR is a technique to achieve relaxation that can be used along with other methods discussed, including guided imagery, meditation, and mindfulness.

Therapeutic Uses of Progressive Muscle Relaxation

Progressive muscle relaxation is a technique used to reduce muscle tension and promote relaxation. It involves systematically tensing and then releasing different muscle groups in the body. This practice has several potential uses and benefits. Here are some examples:

- Reducing anxiety: Progressive muscle relaxation can help alleviate symptoms of anxiety by reducing muscle tension, promoting a sense of calm, and helping individuals become more aware of their bodily sensations and relaxation responses (Bourne, 2020).

- Increased sense of control over moods: The practice of progressive muscle relaxation has been found effective in managing one's mood. By intentionally tensing and then releasing muscle groups, individuals can release tension and experience a greater sense of relaxation, contributing to an overall feeling of control (Bourne, 2020).
- Improving sleep quality: Progressive muscle relaxation is commonly used as a relaxation technique before bedtime. It can help individuals unwind, release physical tension, and clear their minds, making it easier to fall asleep and improve the quality of sleep (Liu et al., 2020).
- Pain management: Research suggests that progressive muscle relaxation may be helpful in managing postoperative pain. By focusing on tensing and then relaxing muscles, individuals may experience a reduction in perceived pain and increased comfort (Tanriverdi, & Kilic, 2023).

Evidence-Based Effects of Progressive Muscle Relaxation

The effect of PMR on abdominal pain and distension in colonoscopy patients was studied using a randomized control design. After a colonoscopy was performed on subjects, abdominal pain and abdominal distension was measured in two groups, one group that was taught to use PMR and a control group that did not use this intervention. The pretest pain and distention scores were similar in both groups, but the experimental group's scores decreased significantly on both pain and distention. Researchers concluded that PMR was an effective intervention and that it helps nurses to "provide better therapeutic care to their patients" (Tanriverdi & Kilic, 2023). PMR also was shown to reduce blood pressure in patients with hypertension, and researchers recommended that PMR be used as a complementary therapy to treat patients with hypertension (Rosdiana & Cahyati, 2023). In patients with coronavirus disease, progressive muscle relaxation was used to test its effects on both anxiety and sleep quality. Researchers found that the average sleep quality scores were significantly different between two groups of subjects after the PMR intervention was used. They also found that there was a significant reduction in anxiety in these subjects (Liu et al., 2020).

Potential Adverse Effects and Concerns

PMR is considered safe and beneficial for reducing muscle tension, promoting relaxation, and alleviating stress. Nurses do need to be aware that like all relaxation techniques, PMR has the potential to trigger emotional release, which can sometimes lead to unexpected reactions. Relaxing muscles may evoke memories, emotions, or traumas associated with body parts, potentially causing distress or emotional discomfort. It is important to approach PMR with self-awareness and seek professional guidance if intense emotional responses occur. Nurses need to be aware of this phenomenon so that they can be on guard against untoward effects of PMR. In rare cases, PMR may paradoxically increase anxiety levels for certain individuals. The act of intentionally focusing on muscle tension and relaxation might heighten awareness of physical sensations, inadvertently triggering anxiety symptoms in susceptible individuals. It is essential to pay attention to individual responses and discontinue PMR if anxiety symptoms worsen.

Nurse Guidance for Use of Progressive Muscle Relaxation

Nurses can support patients with progressive muscle relaxation by guiding them through the technique, teaching them the steps, and providing encouragement. They can create a calm and peaceful environment by dimming lights, playing relaxing music, and ensuring privacy. Nurses can also teach patients deep breathing exercises to accompany muscle relaxation, helping to enhance relaxation and reduce stress. By modeling relaxation techniques and offering reassurance, nurses can empower patients to practice progressive muscle relaxation independently, which can aid in stress reduction, pain management, and overall well-being.

Types of Special Education Required

To teach others progressive muscle relaxation, the type of education required typically falls within the field of psychology or therapy. A solid foundation in psychology, counseling, or a related field would give you the necessary knowledge and skills to effectively teach progressive muscle relaxation techniques. Nurses can teach PMR with more education on stress, anxiety, and the PMR technique (Table 5.2).

In addition to formal education, gaining practical experience is invaluable. This can be achieved through internships, volunteering, or even working with clients under supervision. Engaging in continued professional development, participating in workshops or training programs, focusing on relaxation techniques, and staying up-to-date with the latest research in the field will further enhance your expertise in teaching progressive muscle relaxation.

Table 5.2 Instructions for Progressive Muscle Relaxation

Step 1	Start by finding a comfortable and quiet space where you can conduct relaxation exercises.
Step 2	Begin with deep breathing to center yourself and help participants prepare for the relaxation exercise. Inhale deeply through the nose, hold for a few seconds, and exhale slowly through the mouth. Encourage participants to focus on their breath and let go of any tension.
Step 3	Introduce the concept of progressive muscle relaxation. Explain that this technique involves tensing and then releasing muscles to promote relaxation and reduce muscle tension.
Step 4	Ask participants to identify a specific muscle group they would like to focus on first. It can be helpful to start with either the hands or the feet.
Step 5	Instruct participants to contract the muscles in the chosen area by tensing them as tightly as possible. Hold the tension for about 5–10 seconds, then release and relax the muscles completely. Encourage participants to pay attention to the contrast between tension and relaxation.
Step 6	Move on to the next muscle group, gradually working your way up the body. For example, you can proceed from the hands or feet to the legs, then the abdomen, chest, shoulders, neck, and finally the face.
Step 7	After each muscle group is systematically tensed and relaxed, allow a few moments for participants to experience the relaxation. Encourage them to notice any feelings of warmth, heaviness, or lightness in their relaxed muscles.

Table 5.2 Instructions for Progressive Muscle Relaxation

Step 8	Continue the exercise by progressing through the remaining muscle groups, ensuring participants have enough time to experience relaxation in each area.
Step 9	Conclude the exercise by slowly bringing participants back to awareness, guiding them to gradually open their eyes and reorient themselves to the surroundings.

Breath Work

Breath work, derived from ancient yogic practices, refers to the conscious regulation of breathing patterns. Techniques such as diaphragmatic breathing and alternate nostril breathing stimulate the relaxation response, reduce anxiety, and enhance mental clarity (Jerath et al., 2015).

Therapeutic Uses of Breath Work

Breath work, in clinical practice, is a therapeutic approach that focuses on conscious control and regulation of breathing. It can be used to address a variety of physical, emotional, and psychological issues. By modifying the breath, individuals can activate the body's relaxation response, reduce anxiety levels, improve emotional regulation, and enhance overall well-being. Breath work techniques can also help manage symptoms of chronic pain, promote self-awareness, increase mindfulness, and support trauma healing. Its versatile nature allows it to be integrated into various therapeutic modalities, such as cognitive behavioral therapy, mindfulness-based approaches, and stress reduction programs.

Slow deep abdominal breathing has been a cornerstone of Asian culture and is important to use for self-healing (Deadman, 2018). Many terms are used to describe several types of breathing used for therapeutic purposes, including diaphragmatic breathing, abdominal breathing, and relaxation breathing (Aideyan et al., 2020). Depending on the source you consult, you will be given different instructions for maintaining control over your breathing with the intention of bringing about the relaxation response. In any case, deep breathing interrupts the stress response because it decreases the sympathetic response and increases the parasympathetic response in the body.

Often nasal breathing is recommended rather than mouth breathing. A link has been found between an increase in nitric oxide gas production with nasal breathing. As one breathes through the nose, nitric oxide is produced in the paranasal sinuses, and is then inhaled with every nasal breath (Deadman, 2018). This is important because nitric oxide gas produces many effects in the body: relaxation of smooth muscle fibers such as those in the blood vessels, leading to vasodilation, reduction in blood clotting, actions as a neurotransmitter, enhancement of the immune response, a reduction in inflammation, and enhancement of oxygen flow to the brain.

Breathing for relaxation requires regular practice. It has been suggested that the best way to develop confidence and skill with teaching holistic health practices like deep nasal breathing, progressive muscle relaxation, and guided visual imagery is to learn and practice these skills yourself (Dossey & Keegan, 2022).

Evidence-Based Effects of Breath Work

There is an increasing body of evidence supporting the benefits of breath work techniques. The evidence base for breath work supports its effectiveness in promoting relaxation, reducing stress, improving mental health, and offering potential therapeutic benefits for various physical and psychological conditions. Further research is necessary to explore the underlying mechanisms and optimize breath work interventions.

In one study investigating the effect of breath work on stress and mental health, 12 randomized controlled trials were reviewed for a total of 785 adult participants. The random effects analysis demonstrated a significant small to medium mean effect size and demonstrated that breath work was associated with lower levels of stress than in control groups or conditions. A similar significant effect was seen on anxiety and depressive symptoms (Fincham et al., 2023).

In a second scoping review of breath work interventions for adults diagnosed with anxiety disorders, researchers concluded after reviewing 16 studies that a range of breath work interventions lead to significant improvements in anxiety symptoms in those diagnosed with anxiety disorders (Banushi et al., 2023).

Balban et al. (2023) carried out a study of brief structure respiration practices to determine their effect on mood and physiological arousal. They did find that daily 5-minute breath work and mindfulness mediation improved anxiety and mode in subjects. Breath work was found to improve mood and physiological arousal more than mindfulness meditation.

In a study of a program involving sessions of whole-body movements, postures, and yogic breath work, researchers found a significant improvement in depression, anxiety, and insomnia symptoms in health care workers (Currie et al., 2022).

Potential Adverse Effects and Concerns

Breath work is considered safe and beneficial for health. However, in rare cases, there may be potential adverse effects. Some individuals may experience dizziness, lightheadedness, or hyperventilation due to rapid and forceful breathing. This can lead to a temporary decrease in carbon dioxide levels and alkalosis. Additionally, breath work can trigger emotional responses, and if not managed properly, may cause anxiety or feelings of disorientation. It is important to emphasize that these adverse effects are infrequent and usually temporary.

Nurse Guidance for Use of Breath Work

The role of a nurse in guiding patients in their use of breath work is to provide education, support, and guidance to help patients optimize their breathing techniques for improved health and well-being. Nurses are trained to assess patients' breathing patterns and to identify any issues, such as shallow or rapid breathing, which may indicate respiratory distress.

In the context of breath work, nurses can instruct patients on various breathing exercises, such as deep breathing, diaphragmatic breathing, pursed-lip breathing, or box breathing, depending on the patient's specific needs. They can also educate patients about the benefits of breath work, such as reducing stress, managing anxiety, improving lung function, and increasing overall relaxation.

Nurses may use their knowledge and expertise to help patients understand how breath work influences the body and its various systems.

They can explain the physiological changes that occur during different breathing techniques and help patients develop personalized breath work routines tailored to their specific health goals.

Additionally, nurses can provide emotional support during breath work sessions, as deep breathing exercises can often bring up underlying emotions. They can create a safe and nonjudgmental environment for patients to explore their breath and help them navigate any emotional or physical sensations that may arise during the practice.

The nurse's role in guiding patients in their use of breath work is to empower them to take an active role in their own health and well-being by incorporating effective breathing techniques into their daily lives. Their guidance can make a significant difference in helping patients optimize their breath work practice and reap the benefits it offers.

Table 5.3 Instructions for Deep Nasal Breathing

1. Get into a comfortable position. Uncross arms and legs.
2. Close one's eyes and concentrate on taking a deep breath through your nose and feel the air move into your abdomen. If it helps, place your hand on your abdomen so you can feel it rise and fall.
3. Concentrate on feeling the diaphragm expand as you take a deep, slow breath in. The breath should be drawn in over 6 seconds followed by a brief pause before breathing out for 6 seconds. If this is too long, at first keep of pace of 3 seconds in and 3 seconds out.
4. Keep on practicing for a few minutes and aim for smooth and steady breathing.

It is helpful initially to practice this type of deep breathing three times a day, and when stressful events occur, even if they are minor events, deep breaths can be used. If one practices this technique regularly the technique will be mastered, and thus can be quickly and easily used during more stressful situations in practice.

Nurses can also use deep breathing to manage their stress. When nurses learn to become experts in managing their own stress, they serve as powerful role models for their patients. One source recommends that nurses use this technique during stressful experiences and then in time when nurses encounter stress they will automatically begin using the technique as a matter of habit (Stiller, 2022). Using this technique regularly will help nurses be more comfortable in teaching their clients how to effectively use this relaxation technique when needed.

Types of Special Education Required

Anyone who has pursued education on breath work can teach others to do it, but there are professional organizations dedicated to promoting and educating professionals about breath work and its therapeutic applications. One notable organization is the International Breathwork Foundation (IBF), a global network of professionals that aim to support and facilitate the use of breath work in various therapeutic contexts. Their purpose is "to promote a heart-centered approach to breathwork, its theory and practice, for the expansion of consciousness and for personal and global transformation" (IBF, 2023, para. 2).

We will continue our review of complementary therapies that work on the psychological level, focusing on three therapies that represent the arts being used in a therapeutic way rather than exclusively for aesthetic purposes: art therapy, music therapy, and dance therapy.

Art Therapy

Art therapy allows individuals to express emotions and explore their inner world through various artistic mediums. Mediums might include painting, clay modeling, sculpture, or drawing, to name a few (Natural Medicines, 2022b). Art therapy can be practiced in multiple areas, including schools, private practices, hospitals, or clinics. The creative process fosters self-reflection, emotional regulation, and personal growth. Research indicates that art therapy can reduce symptoms of anxiety, depression, and trauma-related disorders.

Therapeutic Uses of Art Therapy

Art therapy can be particularly beneficial in several ways. First, it offers a nonverbal outlet for emotions, allowing individuals to express themselves when words might be difficult to find (Natural Medicines, 2022b). The art-making process can be cathartic, enabling individuals to release and process their feelings in a safe and supportive environment. See Figure 5.1, Using art as therapy to help others.

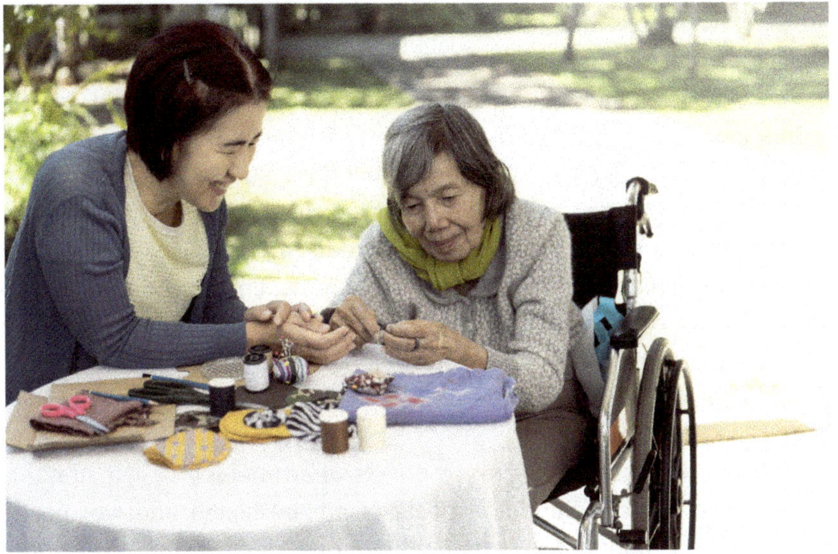

Figure 5.1 Using art as therapy to help others.

Additionally, art therapy can help individuals gain insight into their thoughts, feelings, and behaviors. Creating art provides a visual representation of one's inner world, making it easier to identify and explore underlying issues and patterns. It can also enhance self-awareness and promote self-reflection.

Moreover, art therapy can be a valuable tool for stress reduction and relaxation. Engaging in creative activities can promote mindfulness, allowing individuals to focus on the present moment and find a sense of calm. The act of creating art can be enjoyable and pleasurable, offering a much-needed respite from daily stressors.

Overall, art therapy harnesses the creative process to promote emotional well-being, personal growth, and healing. It can be a powerful and transformative approach to therapy, providing individuals with a unique and expressive way to navigate their inner world.

Evidence-Based Effects of Art Therapy

Art therapy is a therapeutic approach that utilizes the creative process of artmaking to promote personal growth, self-expression, and emotional healing. Numerous studies have demonstrated the efficacy of art therapy in various clinical settings.

In a systematic review of randomized controlled trials (RCTs) and nonrandomized controlled trials on the use of art therapy for managing anxiety in adults, in three RCTs representing 162 subjects results showed some effectiveness of art therapy for pre-exam anxiety in undergraduate studies and possible effectiveness in reducing prerelease anxiety in prisoners (Abbing et al., 2018). Researchers cautioned, though, that no strong conclusions could be drawn and that more study is necessary. Other research has shown that various forms of art therapy can improved symptoms of depression in both adults and adolescents (Natural Medicines, 2022b).

Overall, the evidence-based effects of art therapy demonstrate its potential to improve various aspects of mental health and well-being. However, it is important to note that further research is needed to better understand the specific mechanisms underlying these effects and to identify the most effective art therapy approaches for different populations and conditions.

Potential Adverse Effects and Concerns

Art therapy has been regarded as a safe and effective form of therapeutic intervention for various psychological and emotional issues. However, like any form of therapy, it can also have some adverse effects. Some of the effects that can occur include the following:

- Emotional discomfort: Engaging in art therapy may sometimes lead to the emergence of intense emotions or memories, which can initially cause discomfort or distress. As individuals explore their inner thoughts and feelings through the artistic process, unexpected emotions may arise. This emotional discomfort is considered a normal part of the therapeutic process, but it is important for therapists to provide appropriate support and guidance during these moments (Stuckey & Nobel, 2010).
- Reliving traumatic experiences: Art therapy can involve the exploration and expression of traumatic experiences. While this can be therapeutic and help individuals process their trauma, it may also trigger emotional distress or trauma reactivation. It is

crucial for therapists to create a safe and supportive therapeutic environment, alongside specialized training, to ascertain if the individual is overwhelmed by the therapeutic process (Malchiodi, 2014).

- Artistic frustration: Clients who engage in art therapy may experience frustration if they are dissatisfied with their artistic skills or the outcomes of their work. This frustration can stem from unrealistically comparing their art to the work of others or struggling to fully express their emotions through art. It is important for therapists to address these frustrations by emphasizing the process rather than the end product, supporting self-acceptance and focusing on the exploration of emotions (Wadeson, 2010).

It is crucial to note that adverse effects in art therapy are rare and can typically be managed through the expertise of trained art therapists. The potential benefits of art therapy often outweigh the risks for many individuals seeking therapeutic support (Malchiodi, 2012).

Nurse Guidance for Use of Art Therapy

The role of a nurse in guiding people in their use of art therapy can be multifaceted and supportive. Nurses play a vital role in promoting the principles and benefits of art therapy, as well as facilitating its integration into the overall health care plan. The components of the nurse's role in guiding individuals' use of art therapy are outlined in Table 5.4.

Table 5.4 Components of the Nurses Role in Guiding Individual's Use of Art Therapy

Psychoeducation	Nurses can educate patients about the concept and potential benefits of art therapy. By explaining how art therapy can be used to explore emotions, reduce stress, and enhance overall well-being, nurses can help individuals understand how this form of therapy can complement their health care journey.

Table 5.4 Components of the Nurses Role in Guiding Individual's Use of Art Therapy

Assessment and Referral	Nurses can assess patients' needs and determine if art therapy would be beneficial as part of their treatment plan. They can identify individuals who may benefit from art therapy, such as those struggling with stress, anxiety, or trauma. Upon assessment, nurses can make appropriate referrals to art therapists or incorporate art therapy into their own nursing interventions.
Collaboration	Nurses can collaborate with art therapists to provide comprehensive care. By maintaining open lines of communication and sharing relevant patient information, nurses can contribute to a cohesive interdisciplinary team approach to care. This collaboration ensures that art therapy aligns with the individual's overall treatment goals and needs.
Facilitation	In some cases, nurses can facilitate art therapy sessions or incorporate simple artistic activities into their nursing interventions. While they may not have the extensive training of art therapists, nurses can offer supportive guidance, create a nonjudgmental environment, and encourage patients to express themselves creatively.
Support and Safety	Nurses can provide emotional support to individuals engaged in art therapy, particularly when they encounter challenging emotions or memories during the creative process. They can help individuals navigate through difficult experiences, offering reassurance, encouragement, and referrals to other mental health professionals when necessary.

It is important to note that the nurse's role in art therapy may vary depending on their specific training, experience, and the health care setting they work in. However, by actively participating in promoting and facilitating art therapy, nurses can contribute significantly to the holistic care of individuals seeking therapeutic support.

Types of Special Education Required

To become an art therapist, individuals typically need to complete a specific educational preparation that focuses on the combination of art and therapy. The educational requirements may vary by country or region, but here are some common components of the educational preparation for art therapists:

- Undergraduate degree: Typically, individuals must complete a bachelor's degree in a related field such as psychology, art, or a combination of both. This undergraduate degree provides a foundation in relevant disciplines and may include coursework in psychology, art history, studio art, and human development.
- Graduate degree: Most art therapy programs require a master's degree in art therapy or a related field. These programs often integrate both art therapy theory and practice, providing students with a solid understanding of the therapeutic applications of art and the ethical considerations in the field. The curriculum may cover topics such as art therapy techniques, counseling theories, ethics, assessment, and clinical skills.
- Clinical experience: As part of their educational preparation, aspiring art therapists typically complete a supervised clinical internship or practicum. This allows students to gain hands-on experience in working with clients in a therapeutic setting, under the supervision of experienced art therapists. Clinical experience provides an opportunity for students to develop their assessment and intervention skills while integrating art therapy into their practice.
- Certification and licensure: After completing the required educational preparation, individuals may choose to pursue certification or licensure in art therapy. Requirements for certification and licensure vary by country or state. Certification may involve meeting specific educational and clinical experience criteria, passing a certification exam, and adhering to ethical guidelines set by professional art therapy organizations. Licensure requirements typically involve completing additional supervised clinical hours and passing a licensure examination.

It is important to note that the specific educational requirements for art therapists can vary based on the country, region, or institution offering the program. Aspiring art therapists should research and identify accredited educational programs that align with the requirements of their desired practice location.

Like art, music can also be used in a therapeutic way. Music therapy can be used in diverse ways to improve people's wellness and quality of life.

Music Therapy

Music therapy employs the therapeutic use of music, focusing on physical, emotional, cognitive, and social rehabilitation. By engaging with music, individuals experience emotional release, enhance communication skills, and improve self-expression. Music therapy has shown benefits in populations with depression, anxiety, hypertension, autism, insomnia, pain, Parkinson's disease, schizophrenia, stroke, and dementia (Natural Medicines, 2022c).

Therapeutic Uses of Music Therapy

Music therapy is a field that harnesses the power of music to improve the physical, emotional, cognitive, and social well-being of individuals. It has been utilized in various health care settings, such as hospitals, rehabilitation centers, mental health facilities, and nursing homes, to support patients and promote overall health and wellness.

Music therapy can be provided in several ways. One can be assisted by listening to prerecorded music, and this is one means of eliciting a therapeutic effect. Those who are not trained as a music therapist, but who want to assist people to receive the benefits of music, can plan to deliver music in this way. When a therapist provides music, it is a bit more sophisticated in that the music is used in a definitive therapeutic manner. For example, the therapist may play live music for the patients or assist the patient in creating a song that has meaning for them. Music therapists can design individual experiences with patients involving music that include "improvisation, receptive listening, song writing, lyric discussion, imagery, performance, and learning through music" (Natural Medicines, 2022c, para. 8). Through altering the music pitch, tempo, and melody of the music, different emotions can be evoked. The therapist can also determine the number of sessions needed and frequency. Their overall goal is to bring the patient to a great state of wellness and comfort.

In terms of the mechanism of action of music, multiple explanations have been given. Music provides a means of expressing oneself and is in fact a form of communication. For those who have difficulty expressing themselves due to a congenital or inherited health condition, music may provide a vital avenue for expression and for relationship building that otherwise may be impossible. Music therapy can enhance one's mood, which in turn may reduce anxiety. Likewise, when anxiety is reduced, pain will also be reduced. Music therapy can also provide a needed distraction, and when it is perceived as pleasant, it is understandable why it may bring about therapeutic effects in different patient groups.

Music has been found to stimulate the release of oxytocin and endorphins, and it has also been thought to work on parts of the brain to modulate emotion and motivation (Natural Medicines, 2022c).

Evidence-Based Effects of Music Therapy

The use of music in patient care has been widely recognized for its therapeutic benefits. Research has shown that music therapy can be used as an effective tool to help ease patients' discomfort through difficult procedures or surgery. One study that focused on patients who were postoperative from abdominal surgery demonstrated that relaxation and music interventions helped to ease postoperative pain in this group (Good et al., 2010). In another study exploring the impact of both art and music therapies during stem cell transplantation, it was found that several art and music interventions were beneficial to patients and brought about a feeling of achievement, connection, and enjoyment during stem cell transplantation (Dantanus-Hickey et al., 2022) . These authors stated that art and music interventions uphold the ideas behind holistic and person-centered approaches to care. In a systematic review of the literature on nonpharmacological interventions to reduce anxiety in patients going through medical and dental procedures, researchers reviewed 718 articles accepting 501 experiential trials, which included a total of 50,343 patients in experiments, and noted an overall 71% success rate in reducing patient anxiety when a number of interventions were included, with the most successful being music, cognitive behavioral therapy, relaxation, massage, acupuncture/acupressure, hypnosis, and natural sounds (Weisfeld et al., 2021). Music-related interventions have also been found to have a positive effect on de-escalating agitation in people with dementia with no side effects (Cheung et al., 2023).

These are just a few examples of the evidence supporting the use of music in patient care. It is worth noting that the effectiveness of music therapy may vary depending on the individual and the specific intervention. It is always best to consult with a health care professional or a certified music therapist when considering music as part of patient care.

Potential Adverse Effects and Concerns

Music is very well tolerated. Adverse effects have not been reported in research. (Natural Medicines 2022c). Even so, the following adverse effects are possible and need to be considered when using music to help people. Music therapy can sometimes evoke intense emotions or bring up painful memories, which can be distressing for some individuals. Therapists need to ensure that clients have appropriate coping strategies and support during music therapy. Certain music therapy activities, such as repetitive drumming or prolonged instrument playing, can lead to physical strain or fatigue. Proper technique, warm-up, and monitoring of physical well-being are crucial to prevent injuries. Assessing people for this before, during, and after therapy can help ensure the success of therapy. Music can have varying effects on individuals, and some people may have negative emotional responses to certain genres or styles of music. It is important for therapists to be attentive to individual preferences and adjust the therapeutic approach accordingly. Music therapy may not be suitable or effective for everyone, particularly in cases when individuals have specific mental health conditions or treatment contraindications. Thorough assessments and individualized treatment plans are necessary to ensure the appropriateness of music therapy interventions.

Nurse Guidance for Use of Music Therapy

It is important for the nurse to strive in understanding the benefits of music therapy: One must familiarize self with the positive effects of music therapy, such as reduced anxiety, improved mood, pain management, and enhanced recovery. The nurse should assess a patient's suitability for music therapy by determining if music therapy is appropriate for each patient by considering their medical condition, preferences, and any contraindications. Refer to guidelines from professional organizations like the American Music Therapy Association (AMTA) or the World Federation of Music Therapy (WFMT). The nurse should collaborate with music therapists when they are available. Nurses must recognize that music therapists are trained professionals who specialize in music therapy interventions. Communication with interdisciplinary teams regarding the goals of therapy and the effectiveness is helpful in planning care. Nurses must also collaborate with other health care professionals to integrate music therapy effectively into the patient's overall plan of care. As with all therapies it is important to document the effect of music therapy interventions in the patient's medical record. Nurses should consider striving to use measurable outcomes and reliable and valid measures to determine if there is a substantial impact and effect on the patient.

Types of Special Education Required

The field of music therapy typically requires a specific level of education to become a music therapist. The educational requirements can vary depending on the country and the specific certification or licensure required. A bachelor's degree in music therapy is a common starting point. The American Music Therapy Association (AMTA, 2023) works to both improve the quality of music therapy and improve access to music therapists.

The Certification Board for Music Therapists (CBMT) is a national organization that assists music therapists in becoming board certified. The certification signifies a higher level of learning and dedication to music therapy and demonstrates an advanced level of competence (AMTA, 2023).

A third artform that is also used as therapy involves the therapeutic use of dance. Like music, dance can lift the spirit as it is both therapeutic and enjoyable.

Dance Therapy

Dance/movement therapy (DMT) is defined by the ADTA (2023) as the "psychotherapeutic use of movement to promote emotional, social, cognitive, and physical integration of the individual" (para. 1). This is for the purpose of improving health and well-being.

Therapeutic Uses of Dance Therapy

Dance therapy, also known as dance/movement therapy (DMT), is a form of expressive arts therapy that integrates movement and dance into the therapeutic process. It is used in clinical practice to assist individuals in improving their mental, emotional, and physical well-being. Common uses of dance therapy include the following:

- Psychological disorders: Dance therapy can be beneficial in treating various psychological disorders such as anxiety, depression, posttraumatic stress disorder (PTSD), eating disorders, and substance abuse. By engaging in expressive movement, individuals can explore and express their emotions, enhance self-awareness, and develop coping mechanisms.
- Trauma recovery: Dance therapy has been found to be effective in helping individuals recover from traumatic experiences. The embodiment and expression of emotions through movement can facilitate the release of trauma-related tensions and help process difficult emotions. Dance therapy may also promote self-empowerment, resilience, and a sense of safety.
- Body image and self-esteem: This therapeutic approach can be used to improve body image and boost self-esteem. By engaging in movement and dance, individuals can develop a positive relationship with their bodies, enhance body awareness, and challenge negative body image perceptions. The nonverbal nature of dance therapy may also provide an alternative means of expression for those who struggle with verbal communication.
- Stress reduction: Dance therapy is effective in reducing stress and promoting relaxation. The rhythmic movements and patterns in dance can help regulate the nervous system, increase endorphin production, and induce a sense of calm. This can be particularly helpful for individuals dealing with stress-related conditions such as chronic pain, insomnia, and hypertension.
- Developmental disorders: Dance therapy is often used with individuals who have developmental disorders such as autism spectrum disorder (ASD) or intellectual disabilities. It can help

improve motor skills, coordination, social interactions, and sensory integration. Dance therapy provides a structured and engaging platform for individuals to develop communication skills, express themselves, and form connections with others.

Dance therapy has not only had beneficial effects on motor disorders but also leads to cognitive, social, and mental health benefits as well (Patterson et al., 2018a, 2018b). Dance requires movements and activities that requires both stillness and movement while balancing oneself, turning, and moving at a variety of speeds in a single dance moving forward, backward, and sideways using steps that provide people with the experience for better performances in their tasks in daily life (Swartz et al., 2019). Dance also works on cognitive functioning because people who are dancing need to plan and perform movements, while following the music and various cues for their successful dance. They must remember the steps and have body awareness (Schwartz et al., 2019). Finally, dance is a social activity that requires interactions with others as they perform and encourages the expression of feeling and emotions. Finally, dancers may feel a sense of freedom of movement and enjoyment with the dance (Patterson et al., 2018a, 2018b).

Evidence-Based Effects of Dance Therapy

In a systematic review of the literature, one group of researchers explored the impact of dance as a neurorehabilitation strategy (Aldana-Benitez et al., 2023). They reviewed 25 clinical studies that included dance and outcome measures. They found that there were short-term benefits of rhythmic auditory stimulation on gait, improvements in cognitive flexibility and processing speed, benefits on social parameters, and a reduction in falls in patients with neurological disorders. See Figure 5.2, Seniors having fun at the community center.

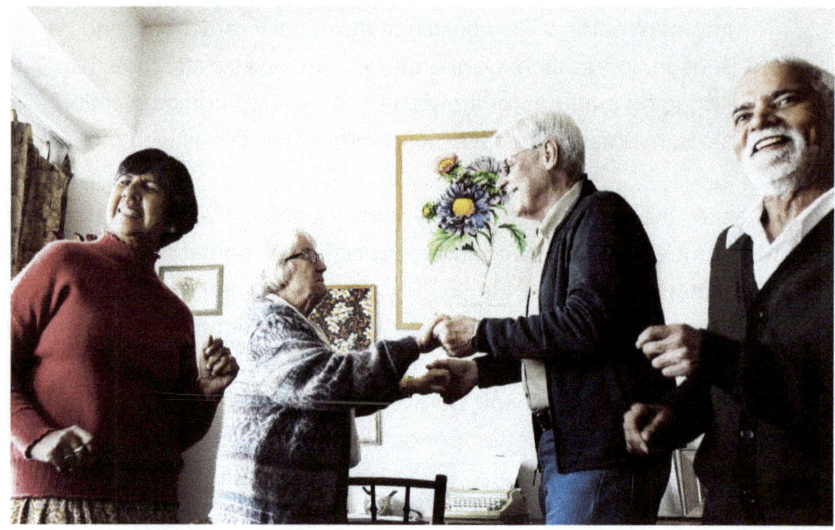

Figure 5.2 Seniors having fun at the community center.

A dance therapy intervention was studied for its impact for children with intellectual disability (ID) at an early childhood special education preschool (Takahashi et al., 2023). Researchers found that dance/movement therapy group sessions for children with ID at the ages 36–72 months led to an improvement in knee extensor muscles and static balance. Maladaptive behaviors were also improved, which led to better enjoyment of the sessions for the full study period (Takahashi et al., 2023).

Dance therapy has been studied as a therapy to help with the symptoms of Parkinson's disease (PD). In a systematic review of dance studies in PD and six randomized controlled trials involving 254 subjects, improvements in gait and balance were noted, and researchers concluded that dance had a positive effect on motor symptoms (Bega et al., 2014).

Potential Adverse Effects and Concerns

Dance therapy, like any form of therapy, has its potential adverse effects. It is important to note that adverse effects can vary from person to person and may not occur for everyone. Here are a few potential adverse effects that have been mentioned in scholarly literature:

- Physical injuries: Dance therapy involves physical movement, and there is a potential risk of physical injuries such as muscle strains, sprains, or falls. These risks can be mitigated through proper warm-up routines, supervision, and adherence to safety guidelines.
- Emotional discomfort: Engaging in dance therapy can sometimes bring up repressed emotions or traumatic memories, which may cause temporary emotional discomfort. Proper guidance and support from a trained dance therapist are crucial to safely navigate these experiences.
- Psychophysiological response: During dance therapy, individuals might experience physiological reactions such as increased heart rate, sweating, or heightened arousal. While these responses can be part of the therapeutic process, they may be uncomfortable or overwhelming for some individuals. Again, the presence of a skilled therapist can help individuals manage these experiences effectively.
- Cultural sensitivity: Dance therapy techniques and approaches may differ across cultures. It is essential for dance therapists to be aware of the cultural backgrounds and values of their clients to avoid potential misunderstandings or inadvertent insensitivity.

It is important to remember that this list is not exhaustive, and adverse effects can vary based on individual circumstances and therapeutic goals.

Nurse Guidance for Use of Dance Therapy

Nurses can play a valuable role in advising patients who are interested in using dance therapy as a form of treatment or self-care. Here are a few suggestions for how nurses can provide guidance:

- Assess the patient's needs: Nurses can start by assessing the patient's physical and emotional well-being to determine if dance therapy is a suitable approach. They can discuss the patient's goals, concerns, and any relevant medical history.
- Educate about dance therapy: Nurses should explain what dance therapy is and how it can benefit patients. They can provide information on the potential physical, emotional, and

mental health benefits of dance therapy and its compatibility with other treatments.

- Find qualified dance therapists: Nurses can help patients locate certified and experienced dance therapists in their area. They can provide referrals or direct patients to reputable resources and organizations that specialize in dance therapy.
- Understand contraindications: Nurses also need to be aware of any contraindications or precautions associated with dance therapy. For example, certain physical conditions or injuries may require modifications or alternative approaches. Nurses can advise patients accordingly and suggest consultations with health care providers if necessary.
- Encourage proper warm-up and safety protocols: Nurses should emphasize the importance of warm-up exercises and safety precautions before engaging in dance therapy. They can provide guidance on proper stretching techniques and reinforce the significance of listening to their bodies to avoid injury.
- Monitor progress and offer support: As patients engage in dance therapy, nurses can follow up with regular check-ins to monitor their progress. They can offer support, answer questions, and address any concerns that may arise during the process.

Remember, while nurses can offer guidance and support, dance therapy should be conducted under the direction of a qualified dance therapist. The nurse's role is to help patients navigate the process and ensure it complements their overall health care.

Types of Special Education Required

To become a dance therapist, a formal education is typically required. A minimum of a bachelor's degree in dance therapy, dance movement therapy, or a related field is necessary to enter this profession. However, some states or countries may have additional requirements or certifications beyond a bachelor's degree, such as a master's degree or licensure.

Dance therapists work in various settings depending on their specialization and the population they serve. They can be found in hospitals, clinics, mental health centers, rehabilitation facilities, schools, community centers, and even private practice. They may work with individuals of all ages, from children to the elderly, and with a range of physical, cognitive, emotional, or psychological conditions. Dance therapists use movement and dance as a therapeutic tool to support their clients' overall well-being and promote personal growth and self-expression.

Hypnotherapy

Hypnotherapy is "the use of hypnosis for therapeutic purposes," while hypnosis is "a state of consciousness with a reduced peripheral awareness and an increased capacity for response to suggestion or instruction" (Natural Medicines, 2023a, para 1).

Hypnosis has also been defined as a "social interaction between two people, one assuming the role of hypnotist and the other taking on the role of hypnotic subject" (Woody & Sadler, 2022, p. 172). During this interaction, each person brings their own interpersonal styles, attitudes, and strategies as related to the role that they take on. As these persons interact, the behaviors that each exhibit may influence and may become entrained, which implies they become "synchronized, coordinated, and mutually supportive or antagonistic—in important ways" (Woody & Sadler, 2022, p. 172).

Sometimes hypnotherapy may involve self-hypnosis in that an individual uses audio-/video-recorded suggestions, while at other times a therapist trained in hypnotherapy may deliver the intervention. Physicians, nurses, and psychologists may deliver hypnotherapy to augment the normal and usual treatment plan for patients. Group sessions may also be used with patients, and these are supplemented with audio-recorded messages.

A hypnotherapy session can be carried out in phases, including a presuggestion phase called induction, a suggestion phase called deepening, and a postsuggestion phase also referred to as a posthypnotic phase (Natural Medicines, 2023a). Hypnotherapists may use a number of tools to test the person's susceptibility to hypnotherapy prior to conducting a session. These tests commonly include the Stanford

Hypnotic Susceptibility Scale, the Harvard Group Scale of Hypnotic Susceptibility, or the Barber Suggestibility Scale.

Therapeutic Uses of Hypnotherapy

Here are a few key uses of hypnotherapy, along with references that you can consult for further information:

- Treating anxiety disorders: Hypnotherapy has been found to be effective in reducing symptoms of anxiety disorders, such as generalized anxiety disorder (GAD) and panic disorder. It can help individuals regulate their emotions and develop coping mechanisms.
- Managing chronic pain: Hypnotherapy has shown promise in helping individuals manage chronic pain conditions, including migraines, fibromyalgia, and back pain. By altering perception and redirecting focus, it can provide pain relief and improve quality of life.
- Overcoming phobias: Hypnotherapy can aid in overcoming specific phobias, such as fear of flying, public speaking, or spiders. It aims to desensitize individuals to their phobic stimuli and replace fear responses with relaxation and calmness.
- Enhancing self-confidence: Hypnotherapy can help individuals increase self-confidence and self-esteem by addressing any underlying negative beliefs or self-doubt. By fostering a positive self-image, it can empower individuals to reach their full potential.

Evidence-Based Effects of Hypnotherapy

Several evidence-based effects of hypnotherapy have emerged from clinical research. First, hypnotherapy has shown beneficial effects in managing several types of pain in a number of studies (Fukui et al., 2020; Taylor & Genkov, 2020; Turner et al., 2023). Different types of pain that have responded to hypnotherapy include abdominal pain in children, irritable bowel syndrome in children and adults, acute pain in both adults and children, chronic pain of various types in adults, and postoperative pain mostly in those undergoing breast surgery (Natural Medicines, 2023a).

Hypnotherapy has also been found to be effective in reducing anxiety. In a literature review by Davis (2015), it was found that hypnotherapy is effective for exam anxiety and is a very effective treatment for state anxiety in those with cancer, surgery, burns, and a number of different medical and dental procedures.

Furthermore, hypnotherapy has shown promise in aiding smoking cessation. A comprehensive intervention review by Barnes et al. (2019) concluded that hypnosis-based interventions were associated with significantly higher quit rates compared to other approaches for smoking cessation.

Overall, these findings suggest that hypnotherapy may be a valuable therapeutic tool for managing chronic pain, reducing anxiety and stress, as well as aiding smoking cessation. It is important to note that while these effects are supported by evidence, individual responses to hypnotherapy may vary. Further research is needed to explore the mechanism of action and long-term effects of hypnotherapy.

Potential Adverse Effects and Concerns

The most reported adverse effects to hypnotherapy include anxiety, drowsiness, dizziness, insomnia, nausea, and headache (Natural Medicines, 2023a). Although others purport that hypnotherapists should assure patients that "hypnosis when used responsibility, poses no risk of untoward side effects (e.g. anxiety, headaches, nausea, dizziness) beyond every day nonhypnotic situations (e.g. taking a test, sitting quietly)" (Lynn et al., 2022, internal citations omitted).

Nurse Guidance for Use of Hypnotherapy

The nurse's role can be instrumental in helping individuals achieve their therapeutic goals through this alternative treatment approach. Hypnotherapy involves the use of guided relaxation techniques to evoke a heightened state of awareness, with the aim of facilitating positive changes in thoughts, behaviors, and emotions. As part of the health care team, nurses play a crucial role in supporting and guiding patients who opt for hypnotherapy.

First and foremost, nurses can provide education and information about hypnotherapy to patients who express an interest in trying it. They can explain the basic principles of hypnotherapy and its potential benefits and clarify any misconceptions or concerns the patient may have. This educational role helps establish trust and encourages informed decision-making.

Furthermore, nurses can assess the suitability of hypnotherapy for individual patients. A thorough assessment involves understanding the patient's medical history, current psychological state, and their specific therapeutic goals. By conducting a comprehensive assessment, nurses can determine if hypnotherapy is a suitable adjunctive therapy in the patient's specific case or if there are any contraindications that should be taken into consideration.

Once hypnotherapy is deemed appropriate, nurses can collaborate with hypnotherapists to develop an individualized treatment plan. They can communicate the patient's goals, preferences, and any relevant clinical information to the hypnotherapist, ensuring that the sessions address the specific needs of the patient.

During hypnotherapy sessions, nurses can provide emotional support and reassurance to patients. They can stay present throughout the sessions, offering a comforting presence and facilitating an environment of trust and safety. Nurses can help patients feel at ease, addressing any anxieties that may arise during the sessions.

Nurses can follow up with patients to gauge their experiences and monitor progress. They can inquire about the therapeutic outcomes, any changes the patient may have noticed, and address any concerns that may have emerged. Nurses can also provide ongoing support and encouragement, helping patients integrate the benefits of hypnotherapy into their daily lives.

The nurse's role in guiding patients who want to use hypnotherapy involves education, assessment, collaboration, emotional support, and ongoing monitoring. By fulfilling these roles, nurses can contribute to the overall success of hypnotherapy as a therapeutic modality, helping patients achieve positive changes in their mental, emotional, and physical well-being.

Types of Special Education Required

In some states hypnotherapy is regulated, while in other states it is not. It is important to be aware of the rules that are required for a hypnotherapist to practice in your state.

There are several respected professional organizations for hypnotherapists that help promote the field, provide resources, and establish ethical standards for practitioners. Here are a few notable ones:

- The American Society of Clinical Hypnosis (ASCH): ASCH (2023) is recognized for its rigorous training programs and standards. It promotes the clinical and scientific uses of hypnosis and provides education, certification, and networking opportunities for professionals in the field.
- International Association of Hypnosis Professionals (IAHP): IAHP (2023) is an international organization that supports the professional growth of hypnosis practitioners. It offers various resources, including certification programs, training events, and a community forum.
- National Guild of Hypnotists (NGH): Established in 1950, the NGH (2023) is the oldest and largest hypnosis organization in the world. It offers certifications, educational conferences, and a range of resources for hypnotherapists.
- Society for Clinical and Experimental Hypnosis (SCEH): SCEH (2023) focuses on the clinical and scientific aspects of hypnosis and encourages high standards in research and practice. It offers conferences, training workshops, and publications to support hypnotherapists.

These organizations provide a platform for hypnotherapists to connect, learn, and stay up-to-date with the latest advancements in the field. It is always a good idea to research and become familiar with the requirements and benefits of each organization before deciding which one aligns best with your professional goals.

Conclusion

Psychological therapies have expanded beyond traditional approaches, with complementary therapies playing a significant role in the promotion of mental health and overall well-being. Mindfulness, meditation, guided imagery, progressive muscle relaxation, breath work, relaxation techniques, art therapy, music therapy, and dance therapy offer individuals a range of innovative and effective strategies to address mental health challenges. As these complementary therapies continue to gain recognition, more research is being conducted to establish their efficacy across diverse populations and settings. Incorporating these approaches into mental health care can provide individuals with holistic support and enhance their overall quality of life.

Discussion Questions for Your Consideration

1. Compare and contrast two or more of the therapies in the chapter. What are the similarities and differences? For example, are the effects of some of these therapies similar? Expound on whether there would be benefits to using more than one of these therapies together. For example, would combining guided imagery and deep breathing have cumulative effects? What does the research show? Include one article on this topic.
2. Consider one medical disorder or challenge and do a review of the literature on psychological therapies for its treatment. For example, in our chapter, dance therapy was identified as having an impact on Parkinson's disease. Complete a 500-word essay reviewing the impact of the psychological therapy on the disorder. If there are conflicting results, please present these. It is important that your review be unbiased.

Experiential Activities

1. Select one of the therapies in this chapter and try it out for yourself. Some therapies that are easy to do on your own include the use of deep breathing, progressive muscle relaxation, and guided imagery. Instructions for each of these are outlined within this chapter. You can use these therapies or any other described in the chapter. Consider using the therapy for three sessions in total to identify if

there are any additional benefits with repetition. After the therapy session(s), please answer the following questions in a minimum of 500 words:

a. Please describe the therapy that you used in some detail.
b. Discuss the immediate benefits (if any) that you experienced and identify if there were cumulative effects that you experienced after using the therapy more than once.
c. Were there any unexpected effects that you experienced with the therapy?
d. What benefits are there with the use of this therapy? Consider doing a small search of the literature and share these.

References

Abbing, A., Ponstein, A., van Hooren, S., de Sonneville, L., Swaab, H., & Baars, E. (2018). The effectiveness of art therapy for anxiety in adults: A systematic review of randomized and non-randomized controlled trials. *PloS One*, *13*(12), e0208716. https://doi.org/10.1371/journal.pone.0208716

Aideyan, B., Martin, G. C., & Beeson, E. T. (2020). A practitioner's guide to breathwork in clinical mental health counseling. *Journal of Mental Health Counseling, 42*(1), 78–94. https://doi.org/10.17744/mehc.42,1.06

Aldana-Benítez, D., Caicedo-Pareja, M. J., Sánchez, D. P., & Ordoñez-Mora, L. T. (2023). Dance as a neurorehabilitation strategy: A systematic review. Journal of Bodywork & Movement Therapies, 35, 348–363. https://doi.org/10.1016/j.jbmt.2023.04.046

American Dance Therapy Association. (2023, August). Home page. https://www.adta.org/

Antall, G. F., & Kresevic, D. (2004). The use of guided imagery to manage pain in elderly orthopaedic population. Orthopaedic Nursing, 23(5), 335–340.

Baird, C. L., Murawski, M. M., & Wu, J. (2010). Efficacy of guided imagery with relaxation for osteoarthritis symptoms and medication intake. Pain Management Nursing, 11(1), 56–65. https://doi.org/10.1016/j.pmn.2009.04.002

Balban, M. Y., Neri, E., Kogon, M. M., Weed, L., Nouriani, B., Jo, B.,Hall, G., Zeitzer, J.M., Spiegel, D., & Huberman, A. D. (2023). Brief structured respiration practices enhance mood and reduce physiological arousal. *Cell Reports Medicine*, *4*(1). 100895. doi: 10.1016/j.xcrm.2022.100895. Epub 2023 Jan 10. PMID: 36630953; PMCID: PMC9873947.

Banushi, B., Brendle, M., Ragnhildstveit, A., Murphy, T., Moore, C., Egberts, J., & Robison, R. (2023). Breathwork interventions for adults with clinically diagnosed anxiety disorders: A scoping review. *Brain Sciences,* 13(2), 256. https://doi.org/10.3390/brainsci13020256

Barnes, J., McRobbie, H., Dong, C. Y., Walker, N., & Hartmann-Boyce, J. (2019). Hypnotherapy for smoking cessation. Cochrane Database of Systematic Reviews, (6). https://doi.org/10.1002/14651858.CD001008.pub3

Bega, D., & Zadikoff, C. (2014). Complementary & alternative management of Parkinson's disease: An evidence-based review of Eastern influenced practices. *Journal of Movement Disorders*, *7*(2), 57–66. https://doi.org/10.14802/jmd.14009

Benson, H. (1984). Beyond the relaxation response. Berkley Publishing Group.

Bourne, E. J. (2020). The anxiety and phobia workbook (7th ed.). New Harbinger.

Creswell, J. D., Pacilio, L. E., Lindsay, E. K., & Brown, K. W. (2014). Brief mindfulness

meditation training alters psychological and neuroendocrine responses to social evaluative stress. Psychoneuroendocrinology, 44, 1–12.
Currie, K., Gupta, B. V., Shivanand, I., Desai, A., Bhatt, S., Tunuguntla, H. S., & Verma, S. (2022). Reductions in anxiety, depression and insomnia in health care workers using a non-pharmaceutical intervention. Frontiers in Psychiatry, 13. https://www.frontiersin.org/articles/10.3389/fpsyt.2022.983165
Davidson, R. J., Kabat-Zinn, J., Schumacher, J., Rosenkranz, M., Muller, D., Santorelli, S. F., & Sheridan, J. F. (2003). Alterations in brain and immune function produced by mindfulness meditation. Psychosomatic Medicine, 65(4), 564–570.
Davis, E. (2015). Literature review of the evidence-base for the effectiveness of hypnotherapy. PACFA.
Deadman, P. (2018). The transformative power of deep slow breathing. *Journal of Chinese Medicine, 116,* 56–62.
Dossey, B., & Keegan, L. (2022). Cognitive-affective strategies to promote resilience and well-being. In M. Blaszko Helming, D. Shields, K. Avino, & W. Rosa (Eds.), Holistic nursing: A handbook for practice (8th ed., pp. 551–567). Jones & Bartlett Learning.
Fincham, G.W., Strauss, C., Montero-Marin, J. *et al.* (2023). Effect of breathwork on stress and mental health: A meta-analysis of randomised-controlled trials. *Scientific Reports,* 13, 432. https://doi.org/10.1038/s41598-022-27247-y
Fish, M. T. (2018). Don't stress about it: A primer on stress and applications for evidence-based stress management interventions in the recreational therapy setting. *Therapeutic Recreation Journal, 52*(4), 390–409.
Fukui, T., Williams, W., Tan, G., & Jensen, M. P. (2020). Combining hypnosis and biofeedback to enhance chronic pain management. *Australian Journal of Clinical Hypnotherapy & Hypnosis*, *41*(1), 3–15.
Good, M., Albert, J. M., Anderson, G. C., Wotman, S., Cong, X., Lane, D. & Ahn, S. (2010). Supplementing relaxation and music for pain after surgery. *Nursing Research, 59*(4), 259–269. https://doi.org/10.1097/NNR.0b013e3181dbb2b3
Goyal, M., Singh, S., Sibinga, E. M. S., Gould, N. F., Rowland-Seymour, A., Sharma, R., Berger, Z., Sleicher, D., Maron, D. D., Shihab, H. M., Ranasinghe, P. D., Linn, S., Saha, S., Bass, E. B., & Haythornthwaite, J. A. (2014). Meditation programs for psychological stress and well-being: A systematic review and meta-analysis. *JAMA Intern Med.,* 174(3), 357–368. https://doi.org/10.1001/jamainternmed.2013.13018
Hofmann, S. G., Sawyer, A. T., Witt, A. A., & Oh, D. (2010). The effect of mindfulness-based therapy on anxiety and depression: A meta-analytic review. Journal of Consulting and Clinical Psychology, 78(2), 169–183.
Hölzel, B. K., Carmody, J., Vangel, M., Congleton, C., Yerramsetti, S. M., Gard, T., & Lazar, S. W. (2011). Mindfulness practice leads to increases in regional brain gray matter density. Psychiatry Research: Neuroimaging, 191(1), 36–43.
International Breathwork Foundation. (2023, August). Home page. https://ibfbreathwork.org/
Jain, S., Shapiro, S. L., Swanick, S., Roesch, S. C., Mills, P. J., Bell, I., & Schwartz, G. E. (2007). A randomized controlled trial of mindfulness meditation versus relaxation training: Effects on distress, positive states of mind, rumination, and distraction. Annals of Behavioral Medicine, 33(1), 11–21.
Jerath, R., Crawford, M.W., Barnes, V.A. *et al.* (2015). Self-regulation of breathing as a primary treatment for anxiety. *Applied Psychophysiology and Biofeedback,* 40, 107–115. https://doi.org/10.1007/s10484-015-9279-8
Jha, A. P., Krompinger, J., & Baime, M. J. (2007). Mindfulness training modifies subsystems of attention. Cognitive, Affective, & Behavioral Neuroscience, 7(2), 109–119.
Kuijpers, H. J., van der Heijden, F.M., Tuinier, S., & Verhoeven, W.M., (2007). Meditation-induced psychosis. *Psychopathology, 40*(6), 461–464. https://ezaccess.libraries.psu.edu/login?url=https://www.proquest.com/scholarly-journals/meditation-induced-psychosis/docview/233347577/se-2
Liu, K., Chen, Y., Wu, D., Lin, R., Wang, Z., & Pan, L. (2020). Effects of progressive muscle

relaxation on anxiety and sleep quality in patients with COVID-19. *Complementary Therapies in Clinical Practice*, *39*, 101132.
Lynn, S. J., Cardeña, E., Green, J. P., & Laurence, J. (2022). The case for clinical hypnosis: Theory and research-based do's and don'ts for clinical practice. *Psychology of Consciousness: Theory, Research, and Practice, 9*(2), 187–200. https://doi.org/10.1037/cns0000257
Malchiodi, C. (2014). Trauma and expressive arts therapy: Brain, body, and imagination in the healing process. Guilford Press.
Mayo Clinic. (2021, March 24*). Stress symptoms: Effects on your body and behavior.* https://www.mayoclinic.org/healthy-lifestyle/stress-managment/in-depth/stress-symptoms/art-20050987
Menzies, V., Taylor, A. G., & Bourguignon, C. (2006). Effects of guided imagery on outcomes of pain, Functional status, and self-efficacy in persons diagnosed with fibromyalgia. Journal of Alternative and Complementary Medicine, 12(1), 23–30. https://doi.org/10.1089/acm.2006.12.23
Mrazek, M. D., Franklin, M. S., Phillips, D. T., Baird, B., & Schooler, J. W. (2013). Mindfulness training improves working memory capacity and GRE performance while reducing mind wandering. Psychological Science, 24(5), 776–781.
National Center for Complementary and Integrative Health. (2023, January). Medication and mindfulness: What you need to know. https://www.nccih.nih.gov/health/meditation-and-mindfulness-what-you-need-to-know
Natural Medicines. (2023a). Hypnotherapy. [monograph]. http://natural medicines.therapeutic research.com.
Natural Medicines. (2022a). Guided imagery. [monograph]. http://natural medicines.therapeutic research.com.
Natural Medicines.(2022b). Art Therapy. [monograph]. http://natural medicines.therapeutic
Natural Medicines. (2022c). Music Therapy. [monograph]. http://natural medicines.therapeutic research.com.
Norris, T. L. (2020). *Essentials pf pathophysiology*. Wolters Kluwer.
Pascoe, M. C., Thompson, D. R., Jenkins, Z. M., & Ski, C. F. (2017). Mindfulness mediates the physiological markers of stress: systematic review and meta-analysis. Journal of Psychiatric Research, 95, 156–178.
Patterson, K., Wong, J. Nguyen, T., & Brooks, D. (2018a). A dance program to improve gait and balance in individuals with chronic stroke: A feasibility study. *Topics in. Stroke Rehabilitation,* 25, 410–416. https://doi.org/10.1080/10749357.2018.1469714
Patterson, K., Wong, J. Nguyen, T., & Brooks, D. (2018b). Dance for the rehabilitation of balance and gait in adults with neurological conditions other than Parkinson's disease: Systematic review. *Heliyon*, 4(3), e00584. . https://doi.org/10.1016/j.heliyon.2018.e00584
Rosdiana, I., & Cahyati, Y. (2023, August). Effect of progressive muscle relaxation (PMR) on blood pressure among patients with hypertension. *International Journal of Advancement in Life Sciences Research*. http://ijalsr.org/index.php/journal/article/view/48
Schwartz, A. E., van Walsem, M. R., Brean, A., & Frich, J. C. (2019). Therapeutic use of music, dance, and rhythmic auditory cueing for patients with Huntington's disease: A systematic review. *Journal of Huntington's Disease.*, 8, 393–420. https://doi.org/10.3233/JHD-190370
Stiller, C. (2022, May–June). Stress management tools to place in your nursing toolbox. Medsurg Nursing, 31(3), 165–168.
Senthil Kavitha, R., & Sasikala, G. A. (2019). Pilot study to evaluate the effectiveness of guided imagery technique on quality of life among hypertensive patients in selected rural areas in Kodaikanal Taluk, Tamilnadu. International Journal of Science and Research, 8(12), 124. DOI: 10.21275/ART20203176.
Stuckey, H. L., & Nobel, J. (2010). The connection between art, healing, and public health: A review of current literature. The American Journal of Public Health, 100(2), 254–263.

Tang, Y. Y., Ma, Y., Wang, J., Fan, Y., Feng, S., Lu, Q., Yu, Q., Sui, D., Rothbart, M.K., Fan, M., & Osner, M. (2007). Short-term meditation training improves attention and self-regulation. Proceedings of the National Academy of Sciences, 104(43), 17152–17156.

Taylor, D. A., & Genkov, K. A. (2020). Hypnotherapy for the treatment of persistent pain: A literature review. Journal of the American Psychiatric Nurses Association, 26(2), 157–161. https://doi.org/10.1177/1078390319835604

Turner, A. P., Edwards, K. A., Jensen, M. P., Ehde, D. M., Day, M. A., & Williams, R. M. (2023). Effects of hypnosis, mindfulness meditation, and education for chronic pain on substance use in veterans: A supplementary analysis of a randomized clinical trial. *Rehabilitation Psychology, 68*(3), 261–270. https://doi.org/10.1037/rep0000507

Wadeson, H. (2010). Art psychotherapy (2nd ed.). Wiley.

Windle, S., Berger, S., & Kim, J. E. E. (2021). Teaching guided imagery and relaxation techniques in undergraduate nursing education. Journal of Holistic Nursing, 39(2), 199–206. https://doi.org/10.1177/0898010120938558

Woody, E., & Sadler, P. (2022). Interpersonal aspects of hypnosis: Twisted pears and other forbidden fruit. *Psychology of Consciousness: Theory, Research, and Practice, 9*(2), 172–186. https://doi.org/10.1037/cns0000229

Xiao, C. X., Lin, Y. J., Lin, R. Q., Liu, A. N., Zhong, G. Q., & Lan, C. F. (2020). Effects of progressive muscle relaxation training on negative emotions and sleep quality in COVID-19 patients: A clinical observational study. *Medicine*, *99*(47), e23185. https://doi.org/10.1097/MD.0000000000023185

Zengin Aydın, L., & Doğan, A. (2023). The effect of guided imagery on postoperative pain management in patients undergoing lower extremity surgical operations. *Orthopaedic Nursing, 42*(2), 105–112. https://doi.org/10.1097/NOR.0000000000000929

Credits

Fig. 5.1: Copyright © 2020 Depositphotos/toa55.
Fig. 5.2: Copyright © 2018 Depositphotos/Rawpixel.

CHAPTER 6

Energy Therapies

> "There has been a revolution in how we perceive the body. What appears to be an object, a three-dimensional anatomical structure, is a process, a constant flow of energy and information."
>
> —DEEPAK CHOPRA

Objectives

This chapter will enable the reader to do the following:

1. Identify varied energy therapies that are used to promote optimum health and care for common health disorders.
2. Discuss the theoretical rationale for the mode of action of various energy therapies.
3. Compare and contrast various energy therapies, including therapeutic touch, yoga, tai chi, acupuncture, healing touch, reiki, and qigong.
4. Discuss common uses for various energy therapies in people.
5. Describe evidence-based effects of various energy therapies.
6. Discuss potential adverse effects to physical therapies in people.
7. Describe the role of health care providers in guiding patients regarding their use of various energy therapies.
8. Discuss the role of health care professionals, types of specialized education required, and guidelines for those who wish to help people with using energy therapies.

Key Terms

Energy therapy: A "broad category of modalities and practices that utilize energy to aid a person in maintaining health and recovering from illness" (Natural Medicines, 2023a, para. 1).

Putative energy therapies: Relate to energy therapies that are not standardized, reproducible, measurements (Natural Medicines, 2023a).

Veritable energy field therapies: Pertain to using measurable energy such as sound waves, lasers, and magnetism for therapeutic reasons (Natural Medicines, 2023a).

Reiki: A Japanese technique that involves the transfer of universal life energy through the therapist's hands (Natural Medicines, 2022a).

Acupuncture: "Acupuncture is a therapeutic modality procedure in which meridian points located on specific body areas are stimulated by piercing with fine needles or applying electric currents or heat. The practice of acupuncture originated in China over 2,000 years ago as a component of traditional Chinese medicine (TCM)" (Natural Medicines, 2023b, para. 1).

Healing touch: A type of energy-based therapy involving the use of light touch, hand placement, and mental intention to balance the patient's energy field (Natural Medicines, 2023a, para. 1).

Therapeutic touch: An energy intervention administered to patients without physical touch. Therapists place their hands over the body and work with the energy fields that surround the body. Therapeutic touch has distinct phases including centering oneself, assessment, clearing the energetic field, and directing/modulating energy (Krieger, 1997).

Qigong: A martial art that originated in China, and those who use it are taught to use their mind and body to control the flow of energy. Mediation, focus, and breathing are essential components of this therapy (Natural Medicine, 2022).

Crystal therapy: Crystal therapy involves the use of gemstones and crystals to balance and harmonize energy in the body for therapeutic effects (Natural Medicine, 2020).

Tai chi: "Involves controlled breathing and slow, rhythmic circular body movements thought to facilitate the flow of internal energy or qi" (Natural Medicine, 2022c)

Yoga: "Uses several exercises involving controlled breathing, meditation, and body posturing" (Natural Medicine, 2024, para. 1).

Introduction

People have for thousands of years used energy therapies (Indian Practitioner, 2022). Energy therapy is a "broad category of modalities and practices that utilize energy to aid a person in maintaining health and recovering from illness" (Natural Medicines, 2023a, para. 1). Energy therapies are used as the therapist focuses on balancing and harmonizing the body's energy system. These therapies recognize the existence of subtle energy fields and aim to promote holistic well-being. The energy therapist's goal is to encourage the flow of energy within and around the body (The Indian Practitioner, 2023). When we refer to energy fields, we refer to putative energy therapies in contrast to veritable energy field therapies. Putative energy therapies relate to energy therapies that are not standardized, reproducible, measurements, while veritable energy field therapies pertain to using measurable energy such as sound waves, lasers, and magnetism for therapeutic reasons (Natural Medicines, 2023a). Putative energy fields are also referred to as biofield therapies.

Energy therapies are based on energy that flows through the body via meridians or around the body through our energy fields moving in and out through energy structures termed chakras. The reader is directed to Chapter 2 where energy field theory has been discussed. The concept of energy fields and various energy therapies have risen from many different places and cultures. We will review a sample of common energy therapies used and referenced in the Western world, but there are countless others used both in the United States and around the globe in multiple cultures.

Types of Energy Therapies

Here are a few energy therapies that are used today:

- Reiki: Reiki is a Japanese technique that involves the transfer of universal life energy through the therapist's hands ((Natural Medicines, 2023). The reiki therapist lays the hands above the patient's body to transfer energy, but energy can also be transferred via distance and with intention. Hands are normally placed in the following positions: "the eyes, back of head, crown of the head, chest or lung area, solar plexus or heart area, abdomen, scapula, sacrum, middle back, lower back and the feet" on average for 2-5 minutes depending on the practitioner (Natural Medicines, 2023, para. 5).

- Acupuncture: "Acupuncture is a therapeutic modality procedure in which meridian points located on specific body areas are stimulated by piercing with fine needles or applying electric currents or heat. The practice of acupuncture originated in China over 2,000 years ago as a component of traditional Chinese medicine (TCM)" (Natural Medicines, 2023b, para. 1).
- Healing touch: This is a type of energy-based therapy involving the use of light touch, hand placement, and mental intention to balance the patient's energy field (Natural Medicines, 2022d). Healing touch is a gentle, noninvasive therapy that involves the use of light touch or sweeping hand motions to influence the body's energy field. Practitioners work to restore balance, relieve pain, reduce anxiety, and support the body's natural healing process.
- Therapeutic touch: This is an energy intervention administered to patients without physical touch. Therapists place their hands over the body and work with the energy fields that surround the body. Therapeutic touch has distinct phases, including centering oneself, assessment, clearing the energetic field, and directing/modulating energy. It is used to reduce pain, induce relaxation, and increase healing in the body (Krieger, 1997).
- Qigong: Qi Gong is a martial art that originated in China. Those using qigong are taught to use their mind and body to control the flow of energy. Mediation, focus, and breathing are essential components of this therapy. There are several types of qigong (Natural Medicines, 2022b).
- Crystal therapy: This involves the use of gemstones and crystals to balance and harmonize energy in the body for therapeutic effects (Natural Medicines, 2020). Practitioners place specific stones on or around the body, believing their energetic properties can facilitate healing, balance chakras, and promote positive changes. Specific crystals are believed to have specific effects in the body.
- Tai chi: This "involves controlled breathing and slow, rhythmic circular body movements thought to facilitate the flow of internal

energy or qi" (Natural Medicines, , 2023, para. 1). Tai Chi was originally developed as a martial art in China and was used for self-defense. There are many different types, but Yang style is the most common. Other styles are Chen style, Lin style, Da Yuan Jiang style, and tai chi ball (Natural Medicines, , 2023).

- Yoga: In yoga, one "use[s] several exercises involving controlled breathing, meditation, and body posturing" (Natural Medicines, 2023, para. 1). There are many different styles of yoga, which use a variety of techniques and intensity so people of widely varying fitness levels can participate. In the Western world yoga most often includes physical yoga poses and breathing techniques (Natural Medicines, 2022c).

Energy therapies are based on the belief that the human body has an energetic system that can be manipulated to restore balance and promote relaxation and healing. These therapies propose that imbalances or blockages in the body's energy flow, often referred to as qi or prana, can lead to physical, emotional, or mental health issues (Energy Therapy Benefits, 2022). One hypothesis is that the most probable mechanism for the effectiveness of complementary therapies based on touch is there is an exchange of energies between therapist and patient due to a bioenergy field around the patients that can be influenced ty the therapist, although this cannot be proven to thoroughly satisfy the scientific community (Micillo et al., 2020).

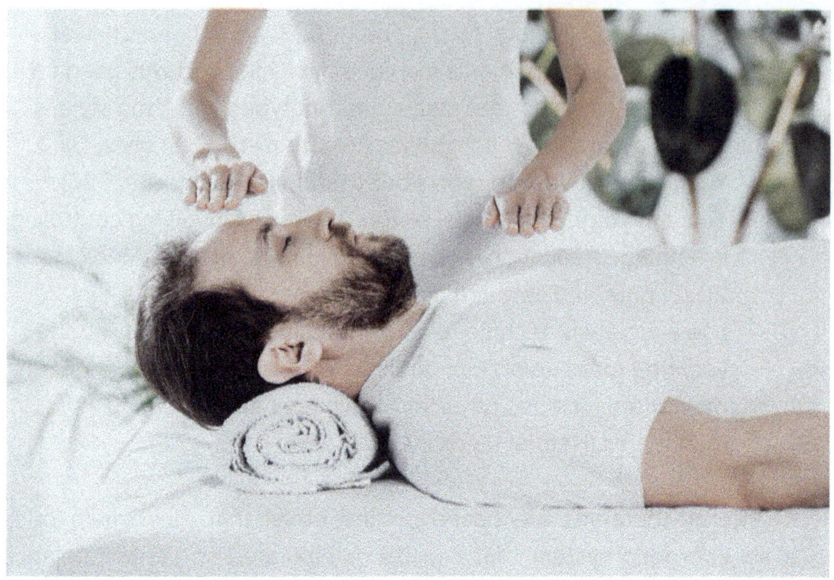

Figure 6.1 Woman doing energy healing.

Each approach has its own specific techniques, but the underlying principle is the same: By manipulating or redirecting the flow of energy in the body, practitioners aim to restore harmony and facilitate the body's natural healing processes. Although the exact mechanisms are not scientifically proven, the theories behind energy therapies often involve concepts from traditional Chinese medicine, Ayurveda, or other ancient healing systems. They suggest that by stimulating certain points or areas on the body, or by channeling and balancing energy, practitioners can help to remove blockages and optimize the body's own healing abilities.

Therapeutic Uses of Energy Therapies

People use energy therapies to optimize their well-being and to help with insomnia, wound healing, hypertension, pain from arthritis and migraines, anxiety, depression, fear, nausea and vomiting, and fatigue (Energy Therapy Benefits, 2022). Therapeutic touch, a nursing intervention, was developed in 1972 by Dolores Krieger and Dora Van Gelder Kunz and has had its greatest effect on pain, anxiety, and healing. Therapeutic touch brings about a state of relaxation within 2 minutes of therapy and does not involve actual touch but rather working with the energy fields around the body.

Evidence-Based Effects of Energy Therapies

The evidence varies depending on the energy therapy you are investigating, but it is important to note that evidence is building that the effectiveness of each of these therapies for different disease states, health conditions, and promoting wellness. Let us review a sample of research on various energy therapies to gain an appreciation for the kinds of effects they may have.

In one meta-analysis investigators examined the effects of acupuncture for chronic pain, with a focus on randomized trials that studied and compared a control group involving acupuncture needling, sham acupuncture, or very simply a no acupuncture control group versus real acupuncture treatments for musculoskeletal pain, osteoarthritis, chronic headache, or shoulder pain. What these researchers discovered was that acupuncture is better than sham treatments or no treatment in managing each of the pain conditions as listed. Researchers also found that the effects last over time, with only a 15% decrease in effectiveness within 1 year. Researchers concluded that referral of patients who have these painful conditions for acupuncture treatment is a sensible option (Vickers et al., 2018). See Figure 6.2, Young woman getting acupuncture.

One group of researchers conducted a systematic review and meta-analysis analyzing the effects of multiple touch therapies, including therapeutic touch, healing touch, and reiki, used in the control of physical and psychological symptoms of patients with cancer. A review of four databases was conducted and found that these touch therapies reduce pain, fatigue, anxiety, and negative mood in patients with cancer but do not influence quality of life or stress (Muz et al., 2023).

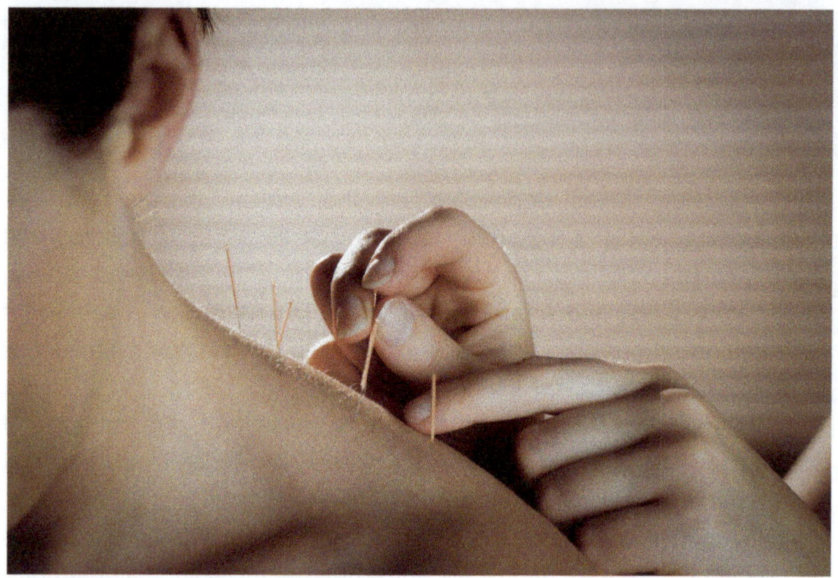

Figure 6.2 Young woman getting acupuncture.

Tai chi is an exercise and is believed to help with energy flow, and therefore this dual action has many benefits to clients. Tai chi has been shown to improve aerobic exercise capacity, benefiting older adults most notably; it also reduces chronic low back pain, improves 6-minute walking distances and pulmonary function in those with COPD, and reduces fall risk in some elderly patients (Natural Medicines, 2022c). Research has also shown that tai chi helps the symptoms of fibromyalgia, improves exercise capacity and left ventricular ejection fraction in those with heart failure, reduces blood pressure, improves sleep quality, reduces waist circumference and body weight in obese clients, and reduces pain and stiffness in those with knee and hip arthritis (Natural Medicines, 2022c).

Yoga, like tai chi, is a movement therapy or exercise. Yoga has been shown to improve the symptoms and quality of life in patients with asthma, alleviate chronic low back pain, have benefits in breast cancer, help with cancer-related fatigue, improve risk factors for cardiovascular disease, help with the management of new-onset depression, improve glycemic control in diabetes, modestly lower blood pressure in those with hypertension, alleviate menopausal symptoms, decrease neck pain and disability, reduce stress, and improve symptoms associated with tuberculosis when combined with antituberculosis therapy (Natural Medicines, 2024).

Potential Adverse Effects and Concerns

Acupuncture does involve puncturing the skin, so bruising, pain, and swelling are a possibility as associated with this energy therapy (Natural Medicines, 2023). More serious effects that are rare but have happened include "acute respiratory failure, circulatory failure, hemothorax, infection at the needle site, pneumocranium, pneumothorax, and death" (Natural Medicines, 2023b, para. 9).

Most other energy therapies do not have adverse effects, but some clients may find that they are very relaxed after therapy, and they should be encouraged to take time to become more aware and alert before operating a motor vehicle or any other activities that could present a safety hazard to someone who is in a highly relaxed state. With the movement energy therapies yoga and tai chi, clients need to be careful to only do the movements and stretches that they are physically capable of doing. A stretch taken too far in yoga could end up with a minor injury such as a sprain. Doing tai chi moves when you already are having trouble with balance or light-headedness could end up in a fall. Other than these reactions, most energy therapies are very safe when provided by a qualified therapist who is taught to observe patients closely and work within their limits.

Nurse Guidance for Use of Energy Therapies

The nurse is in the best position to assess patients and report any untoward effects to therapy. Questioning clients about any injuries, obtaining detailed information, and communicating this to the provider is imperative. Increasing one's knowledge of the effects of each of these therapies puts the nurse in a good position to educate patients and make suggestions for the appropriate therapy for the patient's particular disease state or condition. Although unfortunate, some clients live their life in a state of chronic tension, so when they find themselves in a highly relaxed state after receiving some of these energy therapies it may be perceived as uncomfortable for them. Their response may be exaggerated by the fact that they are used to chronic tension and now are experiencing deep relaxation. It is important for the nurse to be on guard for this reaction if they are providing any of these energy therapies or assisting in an office where they may be discharging patients' postintervention.

Types of Special Education Required

This group of therapies is highly variable. Some therapies are regulated in some states, and some are not. For example, anyone with interest and a desire to help can learn to do reiki or therapeutic touch. Learning involves taking classes from experienced therapists, and there are different levels of education and expertise in both therapeutic touch and reiki therapy. There is no certification for therapeutic touch, and it can be practiced anywhere. Reiki practitioners are unregulated in the United States. In some states though, reiki practitioners must also be licensed massage therapists (Natural Medicines, 2022a). In other therapies, such as healing touch, when there is certification, this involves an education and experiential component before one can be certified. For healing touch certification, a period of mentorship is required. Yoga therapists are educated in classes, schools, or through self-study alone and can be certified or practice without certification.

If you are interested in learning these therapies, it is prudent to take a class first to see if you are comfortable with the therapy. If interested in therapy, research the therapy to see what the requirements are in your state. Many people have made this leap and made a major life decision to become an energy therapist to help people reach a greater state of health.

Conclusion

In this chapter we have touched on energy therapies and discussed how highly variable they are. One thing that all energy therapists have in common is the belief that we are composed of energy and therefore have energy that both courses through and flows around us. By impacting this energy with these therapies, we can positively influence the physical health of human beings.

Little is known about how energy therapies work. Biofield energy cannot yet be precisely measured to the satisfaction of the scientific community, but research can be completed on the effect of the individual therapies on specific disease states and human conditions. Energy therapists should be encouraged to participate in scientific research to further gather data on the effects of individual therapies for specific conditions and disease states.

In the future I anticipate that we will discover the source of the nature of biofield or putative energy fields, but until then, since there are few adverse effects, and many people seem to benefit from these therapies, it seems prudent to encourage their use and of course to continue to research these therapies so science-based recommendations can be made.

Discussion Questions for Your Consideration

1. Compare and contrast two or more of the therapies in the chapter. What are the similarities and differences? For example, are the effects of some of these therapies similar? Also expound on whether there would be benefits of using more than one of these therapies together. For example, would combining crystal therapy and therapeutic touch have cumulative effects? Is there any research on this topic?
2. Consider one medical disorder or challenge and do a review of the literature on energy therapies for its treatment. For example, in our chapter, tai chi was identified as having an impact on osteoarthritis symptoms. Complete a 500-word essay reviewing the impact of the energy therapy on you. If there are conflicting results, please present these also. It is important that your review be unbiased.

Experiential Activities

1. Select one of the therapies in this chapter and try it out for yourself. Some therapies that are easy to do on your own include the use of therapeutic touch, beginner yoga, or beginner tai chi. Instructions for each of these can be found on YouTube, Netflix, TikTok, or multiple other sources. You could also do a search for beginner classes in your geographic area. Some areas of employment have

online access to wellness activities such as these. You may also opt to seek out a therapist for energy therapy if you are so moved. You may use these therapies or any other described in the chapter. Although not required, consider using the therapy for three sessions in total to identify if there are any additional benefits with repetition. Remember to work only within your abilities. After the therapy session(s) please journal using at minimum 500 words and answer the following questions:

a. Please describe the therapy that you used in some detail.
b. Discuss the immediate benefits (if any) that you experienced and identify if there were cumulative effects that you experienced after using the therapy more than once.
c. Were there any unexpected effects that you experienced with the therapy?
d. What benefits are there with the use of this therapy? Consider doing a small search of the literature and share these in your short 500-word journal entry.

References

American Society of Clinical Hypnosis. (2023, August). Home page. https://www.asch.net/aws/ASCH/pt/sp/home_page

Gantt, M., & Orina, J. A. T. (2020). Educate, try, and share: A feasibility study to assess the acceptance and use of reiki as an adjunct therapy for chronic pain in military health care facilities. *Military Medicine*, *185*(3/4), 394–400. https://doi.org/10.1093/milmed/usz271

Gökdere Çinar, H., Alpar, Ş., & Ilhan, S. (2023). Evaluation of the impacts of reiki touch therapy on patients diagnosed with fibromyalgia who are followed in the pain clinic. *Holistic Nursing Practice*, *37*(3), 161–171. https://doi.org/10.1097/HNP.0000000000000497

Graziano, S., & Luigi, C. (2022). Effects of reiki session excluding the variables responsible for the placebo effect on a group of adults. *Alternative Therapies in Health & Medicine*, *28*(1), 18–24.

Energy Therapy Benefits. (2022). Energy therapy: Benefits and uses. The Indian Practitioner, 75 (9), 36.

International Society of Hypnosis. (2023, August). Home page. https://www.ishhypnosis.org/

Karaman, S., & Tan, M. (2021). Effect of reiki therapy on quality of life and fatigue levels of breast cancer patients receiving chemotherapy. *Cancer Nursing*, *44*(6), E652–E658. https://doi.org/10.1097/NCC.0000000000000970

Koçoğlu, F., & Zincir, H. (2021). The effect of reiki on pain, fatigue, and quality of life in adolescents with dysmenorrhea. *Holistic Nursing Practice, 35*(6), 306–314. https://doi.org/10.1097/HNP.0000000000000477

Kramer, D. (2018). Energetic modalities as a self-care technique to reduce stress in nursing

students. *Journal of Holistic Nursing*, *36*(4), 366–373. https://doi.org/10.1177/0898010117745436
Krieger, D. (1997). *Therapeutic touch inner workbook*. Bear and Company.
Micillo, G. P., Nunes Garcia, N. F., Alonso, A. C., Montiel, J. M., & Bastos, M. F. (2020). Implications of therapeutic touch and relaxation massage on aging. *Manual Therapy, Posturology & Rehabilitation Journal*, *18*, 1-4. https://doi.org/10.17784/mtprehabjournal.2020.18.1188
Muz, G., Bilgin, A., Yüce, G. E., & Döner, A. (2023). The Effect of Touch Therapy on Symptoms and Psychosocial Variables in Individuals Diagnosed with Cancer: A Systematic Review and Meta-analysis. Cancer Nursing,10.1097/NCC.0000000000001238. Advance online publication. https://doi.org/10.1097/NCC.0000000000001238
National Guild of Hypnotists. (2023, August). Home page. https://www.ngh.net/
Natural Medicines. (2023a). Energy therapy. [monograph]. http://natural medicines.therapeutic research.com.
Natural Medicines. (2023b). Acupuncture. [monograph]. http://natural medicines.therapeutic research.com.
Natural Medicines. (2022a). Reiki therapy. [monograph]. http://natural medicines.therapeutic research.com.
Natural Medicines. (2022b). QiGong. [monograph]. http://natural medicines.therapeutic research.com.
Natural Medicines. (2022c). Tai chi. [monograph]. http://natural medicines.therapeutic research.com.
Natural Medicines. (2024). Yoga. [monograph]. http://natural medicines.therapeutic research.com.
Natural Medicines. (2020). Chrystal Therapy. [monograph]. http://natural medicines.therapeutic research.com.
Natural Medicines. (2021). Healing Touch. [monograph]. http://natural medicines.therapeutic research.com.
Shang-Jung, W. U., & Wei-Kung, C. (2018). Complementary therapy for patients with limb trauma pain in the emergency department. *Journal of Nursing*, *65*(4), 18–23. https://doi.org/10.6224/JN.201808_65(4).04
Society for Clinical and Experimental Hypnosis. (2023, August). Home page. https://www.sceh.us/
Vicker, A., Vertosick, E., Lewith, G., MacPherson, H., Foster, N., Sherman, K. Irnich, D. Witt, C., & Linde, K. (2018, May). Acupuncture for chronic pain: Update of an individual patient data Meta-analysis. *The Journal of Pain, 19(5)*, 455–474.
Vural Doğru, B., Utli, H., & Şenuzun Aykar, F. (2021). Effect of therapeutic touch on daytime sleepiness, stress, and fatigue among students of nursing and midwifery: A randomized sham- controlled trial. *Complementary Therapies in Clinical Practic*e, *43*. https://doi.org/10.1016/j.ctcp.2021.101322

Credits

Fig. 6.1: Copyright © 2019 Depositphotos/IgorVetushko.
Fig. 6.2: Copyright © 2015 Depositphotos/Wavebreakmedia.

CHAPTER 7

Collaboration With Clients to Integrate Complementary Care

> "If you have knowledge, let others light their candles in it."
>
> —MARGARET FULLER

Objectives

This chapter will enable the reader to do the following:

1. Outline the importance of continually updating one's clinical knowledge of complementary and integrative health programs.
2. Identify exceptional scholarly resources for complementary and integrative care knowledge.
3. Discuss how nurses can use research findings on complementary and integrative care to enhance patient care.
4. Discuss how complementary and integrative health care can be discussed with patients and the public in general.
5. Address reasons some clinicians are suspect of complementary and integrative care.
6. Identify ways that clinicians can find established, experienced, and properly credentialed providers of complementary care.

Key Terms

Wellness: Wellness is a conscious, self-directed, and evolving process of achieving full potential. Wellness is a multidimensional and holistic (encompassing such factors as lifestyle, mental and spiritual well-being, and the environment). Wellness is positive and affirming (Arloski, 2014).

Wellness coaching: "The application of the principles and processes of professional life coaching to the goals of lifestyle improvement for higher levels of wellness" and is an "alliance between a professional coach and a person (or persons) who, through the benefit of that relationship, seeks lasting, lifestyle behavioral change" (Arloski, 2014, p. 40).

Motivational interviewing: "A counseling approach designed to help people find the motivation to make a positive behavior change" (Hartney, 2023, para. 1).

Introduction: Updating Your knowledge on Integrative Care

Staying up-to-date on complementary and integrative care is crucial for nurses and health care professionals in today's dynamic health care landscape. There are several reasons for this. Patients are increasingly seeking alternative methods to complement their conventional medical treatments. In many cases, patients are looking for a more comprehensive and holistic approach that considers not just their physical health but also their mental, emotional, and spiritual well-being. By staying up-to-date on complementary and integrative care, nurses and health care professionals can provide patients with a more comprehensive and patient-centered approach to their care.

Research in the field of complementary and integrative care is advancing rapidly. New evidence is emerging regarding the effectiveness and safety of various therapies. It is essential for health care professionals to stay current with the latest research findings to make informed decisions about the integration of these therapies into patient care. Understanding the evidence base helps ensure that health care practitioners provide safe and effective care. This may seem like a heavy order when one considers the vast amount of learning content that is already required of nurses to learn, but if nurses and other health care providers refuse to stay current on the effects of therapies, they could be denying their clients access to knowledge that could otherwise improve the patients' health status and wellness. Likewise, they may discover that, upon further research, given CITs have no effect at all for specific conditions and they need to make their clients aware of the latest research so that patients' time and energy can be spent on other therapies, traditional or complementary, that have greater evidence for support.

Staying informed about CIT promotes interprofessional

collaboration. Nurses and health care professionals working alongside practitioners of complementary therapies can foster a collaborative and cohesive health care team. This collaboration facilitates a more comprehensive and personalized approach to patient care, combining the best of both conventional and complementary therapies. This type of collaboration is still greatly lacking in the health care arena.

It is the nurse's responsibility to provide patient education and advocacy. By staying up-to-date on complementary and integrative care, nurses can educate patients about the available options, potential benefits, and risks associated with different therapies. Empowering patients with knowledge allows them to make informed decisions about their health and actively participate in their own care.

Staying current on complementary and integrative care enables health care professionals to provide patient-centered care, incorporate evidence-based practices, collaborate effectively, and educate and empower patients. By embracing a multidimensional approach to health care, nurses can better serve patients and improve their overall well-being. The challenge is finding high-quality sources and dedicating precious time and effort to learning about CITs so that information can be located quickly and effortlessly as needed. In earning necessary continuing education units (CEUs) to maintain licensure, consider attending seminars and conferences where CITs and their use to manage uncomfortable symptoms and diagnoses are discussed.

Scholarly Resources on Complementary Therapies

Here are some scholarly sources that nurses and physicians can use to update their knowledge on complementary and integrative care:

- Journal of Alternative and Complementary Medicine: This peer-reviewed journal focuses on research, clinical trials, and reviews related to complementary and integrative approaches to health care.
- Advances in Integrative Medicine: Another peer-reviewed journal that covers research and evidence-based practices in integrative medicine, including herbal medicine, acupuncture,

mind-body medicine, and more.

- JAMA Network Open: This open-access journal includes articles on various medical topics, including complementary and integrative approaches. It often features research and studies related to complementary therapies and their effectiveness.
- The Journal of Alternative and Complementary Therapies: This journal provides evidence-based information on complementary and alternative therapies, including acupuncture, herbal medicine, yoga, and more.
- BMC Complementary and Alternative Medicine: An open-access journal that publishes original research, reviews, and commentaries on various complementary and alternative medicine modalities.
- National Center for Complementary and Integrative Health (NCCIH): This U.S. government agency provides extensive resources on complementary and integrative health. Their website offers research findings, clinical guidelines, educational materials, and the latest news in the field.

It is important to note that the availability of specific scholarly sources may vary depending on institutional access or subscription requirements. Consulting your institution's library or online databases would provide access to extensive collections of scholarly articles and journals related to complementary and integrative care.

Using Research Knowledge to Update Your Nursing Care

Nurses rely on evidence-based practice to make informed and effective care decisions, and this principle applies to all aspects of health care, including complementary and integrative care. When patients are exploring these alternative options, nurses must consider their safety and well-being, as well as their desire for alternative approaches. Here are a few reasons nurses should rely on evidence when making care decisions for patients seeking complementary and integrative care:

- Patient safety: Nurses have a responsibility to ensure the safety of their patients. By basing their decisions on evidence, they can avoid potential risks or adverse effects associated with certain complementary and integrative therapies. Evidence-based practice helps nurses determine which approaches are safe and suitable for their patients' specific conditions.

- Efficacy and effectiveness: Evidence-based practice allows nurses to assess the efficacy and effectiveness of different complementary and integrative approaches. By relying on high-quality research, they can understand the potential benefits and limitations of various therapies, offering patients options that have shown positive outcomes in similar cases.
- Collaboration with patients: By discussing evidence-based information with patients who are exploring complementary and integrative care, nurses can engage in shared decision-making. This collaborative approach ensures that patients are well informed about the available options, empowering them to actively participate in their own care.
- Professional responsibility: Nurses abide by professional standards, which include the commitment to evidence-based practice. By staying up-to-date with the latest research and using it to guide their care decisions, nurses fulfill their professional obligation to provide the best possible care and promote patient well-being.

Ultimately, relying on evidence-based practice when considering complementary and integrative care options helps nurses ensure patient safety, efficacy, collaboration, and professional accountability. It allows them to integrate alternative therapies with conventional care in a manner that is evidence-driven, patient-centered, and conducive to positive health care outcomes.

Teaching and Guiding Patients on Complementary Therapies

Nurses play a crucial role in teaching and guiding patients on the use of complementary and integrative care. Nurses must establish a trusting and nonjudgmental relationship with patients. By providing a supportive environment, patients are more likely to openly discuss their interests and beliefs in complementary and integrative care. Nurses provide education and information and therefore should stay current with the latest research and evidence-based practice in complementary and integrative care. They can explain the benefits, risks, and limitations of different approaches to help patients make informed decisions. Nurses provide care that is tailored to the individual. Every patient is unique, so nurses should personalize care plans accordingly. By understanding patients' needs, preferences, and goals, nurses can recommend specific complementary therapies or modalities that align with their individual circumstances. Nurses engage in a collaborative approach in providing care. Nurses should work in collaboration with other healthcare providers to ensure cohesive and integrated care for the patients. This facilitates the coordination of complementary and conventional treatments while minimizing potential conflicts or adverse reactions. Nurses can empower patients by teaching them self-care techniques that complement conventional treatments. By fostering patient autonomy, they facilitate an active role in health care decision-making and management. Nurses provide follow-up and evaluation. It is important for nurses to monitor patients' progress and evaluate outcomes of complementary and integrative care. Regular follow-up appointments allow the nurse to assess the effectiveness of the chosen therapies and adjust as needed. By employing these strategies, nurses can effectively teach and guide patients in the safe and appropriate use of complementary and integrative care, promoting overall well-being and patient-centered care.

Coaching Clients Who Strive for Wellness

Many nurses integrate coaching clients toward wellness as they provide nursing care in their inpatient or outpatient roles. Other nurses choose to become full-time wellness coaches and may use CIiTs to augment this practice and bring clients closer to wellness. Let us take a moment to consider the topics of wellness and coaching as they are concepts that are so closely threaded into nurses' daily concerns for their clients. Judd Allen, a board member of the National Wellness Institute, surveyed several experts in the wellness field to identify a clear definition of wellness. From this research, Dr. Allen found that participants agreed on the following:

> Wellness is a conscious, self-directed, and evolving process of achieving full potential. Wellness is a multi-dimensional and holistic (encompassing such factors as lifestyle, mental And spiritual well-being and the environment). Wellness is positive and affirming. (Arloski, 2014, p. 38)

Wellness coaching is a field that is about helping clients improve their health behaviors, and it is a relatively new field. Wellness coaching has been defined as "the application of the principles and processes of professional life coaching to the goals of lifestyle improvement for higher levels of wellness" and is an "alliance between a professional coach and a person (or persons) who, through the benefit of that relationship, seeks lasting, lifestyle behavioral change" (Arloski, 2014, p. 40). Nurses coach patients at times and may engage in motivational interviewing. Motivational interviewing is "a counseling approach designed to help people find the motivation to make a positive behavior change" (Hartney, 2023). Nurses may benefit from learning and using motivational interviewing techniques to guide clients toward the use of behaviors that lead them to a state of wellness.

Being Aware That Some Clinicians Are Suspicious of Complementary Care

In the field of medicine, there are varying opinions and perspectives on complementary care. Some health care professionals may hold a certain degree of suspicion or skepticism toward these practices. This skepticism can stem from several factors. Complementary care may involve practices that do not always have substantial scientific evidence supporting their effectiveness. This can lead some health care professionals to question the reliability or legitimacy of such therapies. Some conventional health care professionals may worry about potential side effects or interactions between complementary treatments and conventional medications. Without adequate research or guidelines, they may hesitate to endorse or integrate complementary care into patient treatment plans.

Complementary care practices often lack standardized regulation and oversight, which can raise concerns among health care professionals. This lack of regulation may lead to inconsistent training, quality control, or potential risks to patient safety.

Suspicion or skepticism toward complementary care can have implications for patient care, including limits to integration, communication breakdowns, and missed opportunities for collaboration. Limited integration can result from health care professionals who are suspicious of complementary care and less likely to incorporate these practices into their treatment plans. This could limit patients' access to a variety of therapeutic options that may be beneficial to their well-being. If health care professionals have negative attitudes toward complementary care, it may hinder effective communication with patients who are seeking or already using these therapies. Patients may feel judged, hesitant to share information, or even withhold important details about their health care choices, impeding the development of a trusting health care provider–patient relationship. Skepticism toward complementary care can create a divide between health care professionals who specialize in different approaches. This may prevent interdisciplinary collaboration and limit the potential for combining complementary and conventional treatments to optimize patient outcomes.

To promote patient-centered care, it is important for health care professionals to maintain an open-minded approach and respectful dialogue when discussing complementary care. Collaboration, education, and evidence-based discussions can help bridge the gap and ensure patients receive the most appropriate and beneficial care.

Finding Experienced and Credentialled Complementary Care Therapists

People do not always know where to start when looking for qualified complementary care therapists. When seeking highly qualified complementary care providers to support a client's holistic health journey, several strategies can help locate qualified providers:

- Referrals from trusted sources: Clients can begin by reaching out to their primary care provider and asking for recommendations for complementary care providers. Most clients also seek advice from friends and family members who have had positive experiences with these providers. Their personal testimonials help to identify trustworthy sources.

- Professional directories and accreditation: Clients can explore professional directories such as the National Certification Commission for Acupuncture and Oriental Medicine (NCCAOM) or the American Association of Naturopathic Physicians (AANP) to find certified and accredited practitioners in their area. These directories ensure that providers meet recognized standards of practice.
- Online reviews and ratings: One can check online review platforms and reputable health care websites, such as Healthgrades or Vitals. Reading patient reviews and ratings helps clients assess the quality of care, expertise, and patient satisfaction for different complementary care practitioners.
- Consultations and interviews: Clients can schedule consultations or interviews with potential providers to discuss their goals, concerns, and treatment approaches. This allows the client to gauge their experience, knowledge, and communication style, ensuring a good fit for their individual needs.
- Collaborative networks: Clients can explore collaborative networks where health care providers from different fields work together, such as integrative health clinics. These networks can connect the client with highly qualified complementary care providers who have established relationships with conventional health care professionals.
- Support groups and communities: Clients can join local support groups or wellness communities to connect with individuals who share similar health interests. Within these groups, the client can seek recommendations from members who have successfully integrated complementary care into their health management.

By utilizing these strategies, clients can locate highly qualified complementary care providers who align with their goals, preferences, and values. This comprehensive approach ensures that the client receives optimal care and support on their holistic health journey.Top of Form

Discussion Questions for Your Consideration

1. How familiar are you with complementary care therapies and their potential benefits for patient care?
2. Have you had any previous experiences collaborating with complementary care therapists? If so, what was the outcome, and how did it enhance patient care?
3. Can you share an example of a patient case when you think collaborative care with a complementary care therapist would have provided an additional benefit? How would you envision this collaboration improving the patient's overall care?
4. Is there any CIT that you have concerns about? If so, review the evidence to ascertain whether your concern might be justified. For example, is there evidence to demonstrate that the CIT is safe and effective for all patients? Or, alternatively, is there evidence to show that there are concerns regarding the use of the CIT?

Experiential Activities

1. Role-playing scenarios: Divide into pairs, and one of you assumes the role of a nursing student and the other acts as a complementary care provider. Simulate a patient scenario in which collaboration between the two health care professionals is required. This activity will allow you to understand each other's roles, perspectives, and the potential benefits of collaborative care.
2. Interprofessional case discussion: Consider the case of Mr. Sanchez. He has had arthritis pain for 10 years now and has been on Celebrex during that time. The pain has just increased jumping from a usual pain rated on a 2 to now being an 8 on a numerical rating scale. His X-rays show signs of osteoarthritis in his hands, hip, and shoulder joints. Get into a group of five and each select different complementary care modalities (e.g., acupuncture, massage therapy, or herbal medicine). Your group should research and

present how your modality can enhance patient care in the given case. This activity will encourage interdisciplinary collaboration and expand your knowledge about different complementary care approaches.

3. Patient education workshop: Organize an interactive workshop in which you educate patients or their families about complementary care options. In a small group of no more than four students critically research and prepare presentations on diverse complementary care practices. In the workshop, you can teach patients how to utilize techniques such as relaxation exercises, aromatherapy, or guided imagery. This activity promotes patient empowerment and enables future nurses to incorporate complementary care into their practice. If in person, do a 10-minute presentation using your teaching materials. If online, do a voice over PowerPoint presentation. These experiential activities offer hands-on opportunities for you to gain practical knowledge and develop the skills necessary for collaboration with complementary care providers on complementary care techniques.

References

Arloski, M. (2014). Wellness coaching for lasting lifestyle change (2nd ed.) Whole Person Associates, Inc.

Hartney, E. (November 17, 2023). Understanding motivational interviewing. VeryWellMind. https://www.verywellmind.com/what-is-motivational-interviewing-22378#:~:text=Motivational%20interviewing%20is%20a%20counseling%20approach%20designed%20to,who%20have%20mixed%20feelings%20about%20changing%20their%20behavior

CHAPTER 8

Leadership and Support of Complementary and Integrative Care

> "The purpose of an organization is to enable common men to do uncommon things."
>
> —PETER DRUCKER

Objectives

This chapter will enable the reader to do the following:

1. Identify major professional nursing and medical organizations that support CITs.
2. Identify specialized complementary therapy organizations that support individual CITs.
3. Identify organizations that support alternate medical systems such as TCM, Aryurvedic medicine, naturopathy, and homeopathy.
4. Review examples of educational programs and universities that provide the education of CIT providers.

Professional Organizations That Support Complementary Therapies

Organizational support is very helpful in developing new programs and services. Complementary care therapists, nurses/health professionals, and the public at large benefit from organizations that have made CIT their focus. Several organizations' mission is to support complementary and integrative health care while informing the public of CIT actions, uses, and potential adverse effects. Some organizations are specialty nursing organizations with a focus on complementary therapies, holistic care, and integrative health programs. Other organizations are grounded in educating the public on their view of medicine, such as a focus on educating persons on Chinese medicine, homeopathy, or Ayurvedic medicine. Still other organizations are focused entirely on the development and support of individual therapies such as acupuncture, therapeutic touch, and aromatherapy. We will outline some of this organizational support of CIT use in this chapter.

Organizations That Support Complementary and Integrative Health

These organizations play a crucial role in supporting and advancing the field of complementary therapies, both through research and education. Their missions vary, but they all contribute to the development and integration of these therapies into mainstream health care:

- The National Center for Complementary and Integrative Health: NCCIH is a U.S. government organization that aims to define, understand, and promote the use of complementary and integrative health approaches. Their mission is to conduct rigorous research and provide evidence-based information to the public and health care professionals (National Center for Complementary and Integrative Health, 2024). We have discussed the evolution of this organization's development in earlier chapters.
- The American Holistic Health Association (AHHA): AHHA is a nonprofit organization that advocates for holistic and integrative approaches to wellness. Their mission is to provide resources,

education, and support to individuals and health care professionals, focusing on mind-body-spirit health and the integration of complementary therapies (AHHA, 2023).
- The Integrative Medicine and Health Research Program (IMHRP): IMHRP is a research program at the Mayo Clinic dedicated to studying complementary and integrative medicine. Their mission is to conduct high-quality research, create evidence-based treatment guidelines, and advance the understanding of integrative medicine to improve patient care (IMHRP, 2023). There are many organizations like the IMHRP that have risen from individual health systems to meet the needs of their patients/clients.
- The International Society for Complementary Medicine Research (ISCMR): ISCMR is a global organization that promotes research and collaboration in the field of complementary medicine. Their mission is to enhance scientific understanding, provide a platform for knowledge exchange, and support evidence-based practice in complementary and integrative therapies (ISCMR, 2006).

Nursing Organizations

There are several nursing organizations that support the integration of complementary care into nursing practice by merging these disciplines. Here are a few notable examples:

- AHNA: AHNA is a professional membership organization that promotes holistic nursing, which includes complementary and alternative approaches to healthcare. They provide education, resources, and networking opportunities for nurses interested in integrating complementary care into their practice. (AHNA, 2023)
- ANA: While not solely focused on complementary care, the ANA recognizes the importance of holistic nursing and encourages nurses to consider complementary therapies as part of patient-centered care. They emphasize the need for evidence-based practice and advocate for the integration of complementary care when appropriate (ANA, 2023).

- National Association of Nurse Massage Therapists (NANMT): An organization that supports the incorporation of massage therapy into nursing practice. They provide education and resources for nurses interested in incorporating massage therapy as a complementary approach to patient care (NANMT, 2023).

These organizations serve as resources for nurses interested in learning more about complementary care, connecting with like-minded professionals, and staying up to date on evidence-based practices in this field. It is important for nurses to explore these resources and engage in continuous education to ensure safe and effective integration of complementary care into their nursing practice.

Organizations That Support Alternate Medical Systems

There are several organizations that support and promote various alternative medical systems, such as TCM, Ayurveda, homeopathy, and naturopathy. These organizations strive to advance the knowledge, research, and education surrounding these practices. Here are a few examples:

- TCM: The American Association of Acupuncture and Oriental medicine (AAAOM) is a respected national membership organization. of practitioners and supporters of both acupuncture and oriental medicine (AOM). This organization serves to advance the profession and practice of AOM. The mission of the AAAOM is to "support our members and the AOM. community through education, occupational resources, and legislative advocacy in our commitment to facilitate access to the highest quality of healthcare in the United States" (AAAOM, 2023, para. 2).
- Homeopathy: The American Society of Homeopaths (NASH, 2023) is an organization dedicated to advancing and promoting homeopathy as a holistic approach to health.
- Naturopathy: The American Association of Naturopathic Physicians (AANP, 2023) is the national professional association representing licensed naturopathic doctors in the United States.
- Ayurveda: The National Ayurvedic Medical Association (NAMA,

2023) is an association that supports and promotes the practice of Ayurveda, a traditional system of medicine from India.

Organizations That Support the Development of Individual Therapies

Some organizations are focused entirely on the research and development of individual therapies such as aromatherapy, yoga, therapeutic touch, and herbal therapies, to name a few. Here are some examples for you to consider:

- The International Association of Yoga Therapists (IAYT): A professional organization dedicated to promoting the therapeutic use of yoga. Their mission is to establish and uphold yoga therapy as a recognized and respected health care professional by promoting education, research, and the integration of yoga into mainstream health care (IAYT, 2023).
- Acupuncture: The American Association of Acupuncture and Oriental Medicine (AAAOM, 2023) supports practitioners and promotes the practice of acupuncture and oriental medicine.
- Chiropractic care: The International Chiropractors Association (ICA, 2023) advocates for chiropractic care and supports chiropractors worldwide.
- Therapeutic Touch International Association: In 1979 an organization, Nurse Healers Professional Associates International, Inc. (NH-PAI), was developed to support and promote the energy therapy therapeutic touch, and in 2008 the business name was changed to Therapeutic Touch International Association (TTIA). Now NH-PAI is the credentialing arm of the organization and TTIA (2023) is the membership arm.

Educational Programs and Universities That Educate CIT Providers

There are several types of educational programs that support complementary care providers. These programs aim to provide education, training, and support to individuals interested in pursuing careers in complementary and alternative medicine. Some of these programs are provided by universities and colleges, and others are supported by programs outside of the academic environment. Here are some common types of programs used to educate CIT therapists:

- Degree programs: Some universities offer undergraduate and graduate degree programs specifically tailored to complementary care providers. These programs typically focus on specific disciplines like acupuncture, naturopathy, chiropractic, or homeopathy.
- Certificates and diplomas: Universities may also offer certificate or diploma programs that provide specialized training in specific complementary care practices. These programs may cover topics like holistic nutrition, herbal medicine, or holistic counseling.
- Continuing education: Many universities provide continuing education programs designed for health care practitioners who are already working in complementary care disciplines. These courses can help practitioners stay up to date with the latest research, techniques, and regulations in their field.
- Research support: Some universities have dedicated research centers or departments that focus on complementary care practices. These centers conduct studies, analyze data, and publish research publications, all aimed at advancing the understanding and integration of complementary care into mainstream health care.
- Collaborative initiatives: Universities often collaborate with health care institutions, clinics, and research centers to provide comprehensive care. These joint ventures create opportunities for complementary care providers to work alongside conventional health care professionals, fostering cross-disciplinary collaboration and integrated care.

It is important to note that the availability and scope of these programs may vary among universities and countries. If you are interested in pursuing a career in complementary care, I recommend researching specific universities or institutions that offer programs aligned with your interests and goals.

Conclusion

In this chapter several organizations were outlined for your consideration. There is much support for complementary therapy use, and these organizations continue to grow in numbers and funding so that CITs can be properly supported and used most effectively for the evidence-based management of people's health care.

Discussion Questions for Your Consideration

1. How can incorporating education and training in complementary care modalities enhance the nursing profession and improve patient outcomes?
2. What role does organizational leadership play in promoting the integration of complementary care within health care institutions, and how can nursing professionals contribute to this process?
3. In what ways can you as a nursing student actively advocate for the inclusion of complementary care education within nursing curricula and ensure its recognition within health care organizations?

Experiential Activities

1. Role play–based simulation: Get into a group of four. Consider this patient: Ashley Jones has had fibromyalgia syndrome for 5 years, leaving her with osteoarthritis pain, multiple points of tender point pain throughout her body, and severe fatigue. Organize a role-playing scenario in which each of you take on the roles of different health care professionals, including nurses, doctors, complementary therapists, and administrators, to discuss how her care and others like her might best be managed. You can learn about the challenges and benefits of organizational support for these therapies.
2. Panel discussion with complementary therapists: Invite and organize complementary therapists from different disciplines to participate in

a panel discussion with nursing students. The therapists can talk about their experiences working within health care organizations and their collaboration with nursing staff. This activity will provide insights into the types of support and resources necessary for the successful integration of complementary therapies. Students can also interact with therapists and ask questions to gain a deeper understanding of the organizational dynamics.

3. Site visit to an integrative health care center: Organize a field trip to an integrative health care center that supports complementary therapies. You can tour the facility, observe therapy sessions, and engage in discussions with health care professionals working there. This activity will expose you to the day-to-day operations of an organization that offers complementary therapies, providing a practical understanding of how such therapies are integrated into patient care. Students can learn about the administrative processes, collaboration between health care professionals, and the positive impact of organizational support.

By engaging in these experiential activities, you can gain an appreciation for the importance of organizational support in facilitating the inclusion and effectiveness of complementary therapies within health care settings.

References

American Association of Acupuncture and Oriental Medicine. (2023, October). Home page. https://www.aaaomonline.org/

American Holistic Health Association. (2023, October). Home page. https://ahha.org/

American Nurses Association. (2023, October). Home page. https://www.nursingworld.org/ana/

American Society for Naturopathic Physicians. (2023, October). Home page. https://naturopathic.org/

Integrative Medicine and Health. (2023, October). Home page. https://www.mayoclinic.org/departments-centers/integrative-medicine-health/sections/overview/ovc-20464567

International Association of Yoga Therapists. (2023, October). About us. https://www.iayt.org/page/AboutLanding

International Chiropractors Association. (2023, October). Home page. https://www.chiropractic.org/

International Society for Complementary Medicine Research. (2006). https://www.researchgate.net/publication/7229204_

National Association of Nurse Massage Therapists. (2023, October). The power of touch. http://www.nanmt.org/index-1philosophy.html

National Ayurvedic Medical Association. (2023, October). Home page. https://www.ayurvedanama.org/

The National Center for Complementary and Integrative Health. (2024). About NCCIH. https://www.nccih.nih.gov/about.

North The American Society of Homeopaths. (2023, October). Home page. https://homeopathy.org/

Therapeutic Touch International Association (2023, October). Home page. https://therapeutictouch.org/

CHAPTER 9

Charting the Future for Complementary and Integrative Care

> "Strength and growth come only through continuous effort and struggle."
>
> —NAPOLEON HILL, AUTHOR

Objectives

This chapter will enable the reader to do the following:

1. Describe the epistemology of complementary and integrative care and share how new knowledge will continue to evolve, overlapping with traditional models of care.
2. Relay the importance of encouraging the education of CIT providers.
3. Identify that traditional providers need to cultivate their own knowledge of CIT.
4. Discuss the need for the continued development of high-quality resources of CIT knowledge for both clinicians and all members of the public.
5. Discuss the need for the regulation of some CIT services and programs.

Introduction: The Epistemology of Complementary Care Knowledge Development

In this chapter we will revisit the historical development of complementary and integrative care development, but with an emphasis of CIT knowledge development in the United States, and discuss key events, influential figures, and the evolution of attitudes and acceptance toward this form of health care.

The roots of complementary and integrative care in the United States can be traced back to the early 19th century when various healing systems such as homeopathy, naturopathy, and chiropractic emerged. These alternative approaches challenged the dominant allopathic model of health care and provided alternative methods for addressing illness and maintaining health. Early practitioners like Samuel Hahnemann, the founder of homeopathy, and Benedict Lust, credited as the father of naturopathy, laid the groundwork for the future development of these disciplines.

The development of complementary and integrative care knowledge gained momentum during the mid-20th century. This shift toward mainstream acceptance can be attributed to several factors, including dissatisfaction with the side effects of pharmaceutical drugs, the desire for more patient-centered care, and increasing interest in natural and holistic health approaches. The counterculture movements of the 1960s and 1970s further fueled the demand for alternatives to conventional medicine, leading to the popularization of practices such as acupuncture, yoga, and meditation. People began to realize that they had some control over their own health and wellness.

Several influential organizations played a crucial role in advancing the knowledge and acceptance of complementary and integrative care in the United States. The establishment of the NCCIH in 1998 within the National Institutes of Health (NIH) was a significant milestone. The NCCIH supports research and provides evidence-based information on complementary and integrative health practices to both health care professionals and the public. Additionally, the creation of the Consortium of Academic Health Centers for Integrative Medicine further legitimized and integrated complementary care within conventional medical education.

The rise of patient-centered care as a guiding principle in health care paved the way for the integration of complementary and integrative care. This approach recognizes the importance of treating the whole person rather than solely focusing on the disease or symptoms. Furthermore, the emphasis on evidence-based practices has played a crucial role in the development of complementary and integrative care knowledge. Rigorous scientific research and clinical trials have helped establish the effectiveness and safety of many complementary therapies, promoting wider acceptance by health care professionals and the public.

Complementary and integrative care continues to gain acceptance in the United States health care system. Many major medical centers now offer integrative medicine programs, and an increasing number of health insurance plans cover selected complementary therapies. The ongoing research in fields such as mind-body medicine, acupuncture, herbal medicine, and nutrition continues to contribute to the advancement of complementary and integrative care knowledge.

The historical development of complementary and integrative care knowledge in the United States has been marked by a shift from marginalization to increased acceptance and integration. Influential figures, organizations, and evolving attitudes toward health care have contributed to this transformation. As the healthcare landscape evolves, it is essential to continue supporting rigorous research, education, and collaboration between conventional and complementary care practitioners to further promote patient well-being and provide comprehensive health care options.

Education of Complementary Care Therapists

Complementary care therapists encompass a diverse range of practices that aim to support overall well-being, often in conjunction with mainstream medical treatments. These therapists receive education and training specific to their chosen therapy, and the nature of their education can vary depending on the therapy they practice.

Some therapies, such as massage therapy or acupuncture, require formal education and licensing. Massage therapists typically complete programs that may range from a few months to a couple of years, involving hands-on training in techniques, anatomy, and physiology. Similarly, acupuncturists undergo specialized training that involves learning about traditional Chinese medicine principles, diagnostic techniques, and the practice of inserting needles at specific points in the body.

Other complementary care therapies, like aromatherapy or reiki, may not require formal licensing or extensive formal education. However, practitioners typically undertake specific training programs or certifications to gain in-depth knowledge and skills. For instance, aromatherapists may attend workshops or courses to learn about the properties, uses, and safety considerations of essential oils. Reiki practitioners often undergo a series of attunements or levels of training to become proficient in this energy healing modality.

Different therapy modalities also differ in terms of their educational pathways. For example, chiropractors undergo extensive education, earning a Doctor of Chiropractic degree, which typically involves 4 years of postgraduate education. Naturopathic doctors complete a rigorous 4-year program at accredited naturopathic medical schools to learn various natural healing methods and diagnostics.

Overall, while some complementary care therapists may have formal educational requirements and licensing processes, others may rely more on specialized training, certifications, or apprenticeships. Regardless of the therapy, ongoing professional development and staying updated with the latest research and practices are considered essential for any complementary care therapist.

Importance of Education of Providers on Complementary Care Therapies

It is essential to educate complementary care therapists for several reasons. First, proper education ensures therapists have the knowledge and skills required to provide safe and effective care to patients. Education equips therapists with a deep understanding of various complementary therapies, enabling them to tailor treatments to individual needs. Additionally, education helps therapists stay current with the latest research and developments in the field, allowing them to provide evidence-based care. Lastly, by highlighting ethical considerations, communication skills, and professional boundaries, education ensures therapists maintain exacting standards of practice and uphold the well-being and trust of their patients.

Development of CIT Knowledge and Resources

Over the past century, there has been a significant development and recognition of complementary care resources. One notable development in complementary care resources has been the emergence of professional organizations and associations dedicated to promoting and advancing the field. These organizations have facilitated the sharing of knowledge, research, and best practices among practitioners, creating a more cohesive and robust framework for complementary care, as discussed in Chapter 8. Additionally, the internet and advancements in technology have played a crucial role in the accessibility of complementary care resources. Online platforms, websites, and social media have made it easier for individuals to access information, connect with experts, and find resources related to complementary care.

There are several specific complementary care resources available today for individuals seeking to increase their understanding and knowledge. Here are a few examples:

- Books and literature: A vast array of books have been published on various forms of complementary care, such as acupuncture, herbal medicine, meditation, and more. These books provide comprehensive information and practical guidance.
- Online courses and webinars: Many organizations, institutions, and individual practitioners offer online courses and webinars to educate individuals about several aspects of complementary care. These interactive resources often cover specific techniques, approaches, or conditions.
- Research journals: Academic journals focusing on complementary care publish studies, research findings, and evidence-based articles. Such journals contribute to the development of knowledge and facilitate ongoing discourse in the field.
- Podcasts and audio resources: Numerous podcasts and audio recordings are available, featuring conversations with experts,

interviews, and discussions about complementary care modalities.
- Community workshops and seminars: Local communities often organize workshops, seminars, and events that aim to introduce and educate individuals about complementary care practices. These events provide opportunities for hands-on experiences, question-and-answer sessions, and practical demonstrations.

While complementary care has gained recognition and acceptance, it is important to consult with qualified health care professionals and ensure any chosen approach aligns with an individual's specific health care needs.

Regulation of Complementary Care Therapies

In the United States, complementary care, which includes various practices and therapies such as acupuncture, chiropractic care, and herbal medicine, is regulated differently from conventional medicine. While there is no specific comprehensive set of regulations that applies to complementary care at the federal level, several factors influence the practice and availability of these treatments.

Regulations pertaining to complementary care primarily fall under state jurisdiction, resulting in variations from one state to state. Some states have established regulatory boards to oversee and license practitioners of specific complementary therapies. For example, chiropractors are regulated by state chiropractic boards, while acupuncturists may be governed by state acupuncture boards.

Insurance coverage for complementary care is another significant aspect affected by regulations. The level of coverage and reimbursement often varies based on state regulations and specific insurance plans. Some states have laws mandating insurance coverage for certain complementary therapies, while others provide limited or no coverage. Additionally, insurance companies may have their own policies regarding reimbursement for complementary care.

Another important consideration is the regulation of dietary supplements and herbal medicines. The DSHEA of 1994 established guidelines for the regulation of dietary supplements, including vitamins, minerals, and herbal products. Under DSHEA, supplements are regulated as food products rather than drugs. This means that manufacturers are responsible for ensuring the safety and labeling accuracy of their products, but they are not required to prove their efficacy before marketing them.

The regulation of complementary care is an ongoing process, and there are ongoing debates concerning the appropriate level of regulation. Some argue for tighter regulation to ensure patient safety and standardization, while others advocate for a more hands-off approach to allow for individual autonomy and access to a wider range of treatment options.

Overall, the regulatory landscape for complementary care in the United States varies by state and specific therapy, and it is important to stay informed about the regulations in your area and consult with licensed practitioners for the best advice on availability, insurance coverage, and safety considerations.

Conclusion

In this chapter we discussed the emergence of CITs as separate areas of knowledge development. The importance of education for the public was discussed, with some varied options as sources of education outlined. The proper education of CIT therapists was emphasized. Regulation of therapies is an important topic of consideration and is at this time highly variable depending both on the specific therapy and the state in which one lives. There is one thing for certain: CIT development is still very much in progress, and research continues to forge new avenues for care and applications for specific complementary therapies.

Discussion Questions for Your Consideration

1. Why is it essential for nurses to educate themselves and other providers on complementary care practices?
2. How can nurses effectively promote the integration of complementary care into conventional medical practice by educating themselves and other health care providers?
3. Locate a current educational resource (5 years or less) on a

complementary care therapy of your choice and critique it based on how the resource addresses the therapy's evidence-based practice support, safety considerations, and cultural relevancy? Does the source include any tools for nurses or providers in educating their clients on the therapy? Submit your analysis of these questions and include either the link or the resource citation for the source.

Experiential Activities

Case Study: Sarah's journey with reiki therapy

Background: Sarah, a 45-year-old woman, has been battling chronic pain and stress due to her busy work schedule and personal responsibilities. She has tried various conventional treatments and medications, but they only provided temporary relief. Seeking additional support, Sarah decided to explore complementary therapies and discovered reiki, a form of energy healing.

Reiki therapy: Sarah began receiving regular reiki sessions from a trained practitioner. This therapy involves the gentle laying on of hands to channel healing energy throughout the patient's body. The goal is to balance energy, promote relaxation, and facilitate the body's natural healing processes.

Benefits experienced:

- Reduced pain levels: Over time, Sarah noticed a significant reduction in her chronic pain levels. The calming nature of reiki helped alleviate tension, relax her muscles, and promote a sense of well-being.
- Improved sleep quality: Sarah had been struggling with insomnia for years, but after several Reiki sessions, she experienced a more restful and rejuvenating sleep. This enhanced sleep quality contributed to her overall improved well-being and energy levels.
- Reduced stress and anxiety: Reiki therapy had a profound impact on Sarah's stress and anxiety levels. Regular treatments

allowed her to unwind, release emotional tension, and discover a newfound sense of inner peace.

- Enhanced emotional well-being: Reiki sessions facilitated emotional healing and provided Sarah with a supportive environment to address past traumas and regain emotional balance. This newfound emotional well-being positively impacted her overall quality of life.

Discussion Questions for Nursing Students:

1. What is Reiki therapy, and how does it differ from traditional medical interventions?
2. What are the potential benefits of incorporating complementary therapies like Reiki into nursing care plans?
3. How can nurses educate patients about the benefits and potential risks of complementary therapies?
4. What are the ethical considerations when discussing and promoting complementary therapies in a healthcare setting?
5. How can nurses collaborate with complementary therapy practitioners to ensure holistic and patient-centered care delivery?
6. What research evidence supports the utilization of complementary therapies in nursing practice?
7. How can nurses inform and educate patients about the importance of seeking evidence-based complementary therapies rather than falling victim to misinformation or scams?

By discussing these questions, nursing students can gain insights into the benefits of complementary therapies like Reiki and their role in enhancing patient care. Additionally, exploring these topics will foster understanding and equip students with the knowledge to educate patients about the safe integration of complementary therapies into their healthcare journey.

CHAPTER 10

Exemplars of Integrative Care

"The reality is that the only way change comes is when you lead by example."

—ANNE WOJCICKI

Objectives

This chapter will enable the reader to do the following:

1. Identify integrative care programs that have been used for varied clinical problems with success both in health centers and community agencies.
2. Discuss the structures that have been used to integrate CIT throughout time and in different clinical and community settings.
3. Discuss qualities of successful CIT programs.

Introduction

It is a challenge to be charged with starting any new line of services such as complementary or integrative care within a health care system. In 1998 this author was given the opportunity to start a freestanding hospital-based complementary care center (CCC) and to integrate complementary care therapies in a rural hospital setting. There were few CC services available in the local community at the time. Without having many centers to model, a team developed the center based on logic, reason, evidence-based research support, and previous experience with providing health care services for the public. In this chapter we will begin by discussing the practical steps that were taken to start up the CCC to help others who are tasked with this responsibility.

A core of staff members was brought on to handle the task of creating a CCC. A medical director was appointed and emphasized the need to gather evidence regarding each therapy's effectiveness. This author served as director of complementary care and managed the daily affairs of providing CITs offsite from the hospital and handled integration of therapies into care at the hospital. A yoga director who had some prior success in bringing in interested clients within the community was also hired and managed the yoga studio and hiring of additional yoga teachers. A hospital administrator worked with each of the full-time associates to get things started and to organize the financial support for the venture. All other associates worked as independent contractors, and the following therapists were brought on board: an herbalist, aromatherapist, massage therapist, therapeutic touch practitioner, craniosacral therapist, reflexologist, and a medical acupuncturist. Attention was given to finding the most qualified and experienced therapists possible as well as to governmental regulations of some therapies, such as massage therapy, in the region. Investments were made in sending some associates to national seminars to get abreast of the latest information on CIT in the United States. Policies regarding managing payroll and policies for payment of independent contractors were developed. Monthly meetings were held to update all full-time associates and independent contractors, to share new developments, and to report on regular changes.

An offsite office space was converted to a therapeutic place for people to gather. The thought regarding being offsite from the hospital was that many persons who need complementary care might choose to go somewhere other than a hospital for this care. The primary administrator selected a space in the community that was already contracted to be rented previously by the hospital and was not currently being used. It included a large yoga studio, a front office, a spa-like shower and locker facility, a juice bar, and many rooms where individual therapies could be provided. Attention was given to aesthetics with the inclusion of art, music, and a small library of books that could be checked out by visitors. Attention was also given to practical elements, including incorporating live plants and arranging for their care; providing aromatherapy via diffusers for special events and during therapy sessions; and purchasing massage tables, a reflexology chair, massage therapy oils, a device to keep towels moist and warm for massage therapy, desks, chairs, and office furniture. Organic cleaning was arranged for and sterilization of some of the supplies for acupuncture had to be organized. Massage therapy oils, towels, robes, slippers for the locker room, acupuncture needles/supplies, aromatherapy, and refreshments for the juice bar were ordered.

As the CCC was developed, this author became aware that people in this rural community had very little knowledge about complementary and integrative care. Many clients coming to the CCC for therapies did not know which therapy could be most effective to manage their condition or symptoms. It was decided to offer an initial consultation to review clients' health concerns and help them select a therapy that had documented evidence-based effects, as demonstrated in prior research. As the director with clinical, complementary care, and research experience, I was poised to complete these initial meetings with potential clients. Clients were then funneled to therapists to receive CIT for their conditions. Clients reported a whole gamut of health problems, including back pain, carpal tunnel pain, infertility, depression, anxiety, and arthritis, to name a few. Consistent with prior research findings, many of these clients did not get relief from their problems with conventional medical care and sought out complementary care. In addition, other clients were simply searching for a higher level of well-being by participating in the many diverse types and levels of yoga classes that the yoga director provided, in therapeutic free-form dancing classes, or coming to the CCC for regular massage.

As the CCC was developed, a focus on communications with the public and local community was designed and executed. Informational pamphlets on each of the therapies were created. A 10-minute informational commercial was produced and presented on local television. The local newspaper produced stories on many of the education sessions and events that took place at the CCC. Seminars were presented both at the CCC and at the local hospital. One seminar was designed specifically to inform physicians about the various therapies that were provided and how they might be helpful for clients with different symptoms and diagnoses. A mind-body interest group was established for anyone who wanted to attend monthly meetings and learn about CIT use and wholistic health topics. A CCC newsletter was also distributed at the CCC and within the associated health center to both inform and garner interest from members of the local community.

The rural health care system dedicated resources to the development of this CCC and increased the local communities' use of these services. As the line of services were developed and rolled out therapists began to work with hospital unit leaders in integrating complementary care services with traditional medical care for positive patient outcomes. Integration started out with aromatherapy use for the OR waiting areas focusing on lavender use for relaxation of visitors to the operating room. Policies for integration of CITs into the hospital setting were developed, starting with therapeutic touch and bedside yoga policies. Much education of health care leaders within the organization was required to assist them in seeing the significance of CIT use within the hospital.

Complementary and integrative care centers have been opening around the country since this time, and we have learned much about how to best provide CITs to the public. Considering some common structures for CITs will help to further understand how this is best accomplished. In this next section we will review the common structure of complementary and integrative programs.

Structures of Complementary and Integrative Care Programs

Integrative health programs are typically organized or structured to provide a comprehensive approach to health care and incorporate both conventional and complementary therapies. While the specifics may vary, here are some common features and principles often found in integrative health programs:

- Multidisciplinary approach: Integrative health programs bring together health care professionals from various disciplines, such as medical doctors, naturopathic doctors, nutritionists, physical therapists, and mental health professionals. This collaborative approach allows for a more holistic assessment and treatment plan.
- Patient-centered care: These programs prioritize the needs and goals of the individual patient. The focus is on treating the whole person rather than just the symptoms or conditions they present. Patients are actively involved in decision-making and encouraged to take responsibility for their health.
- Personalized treatment plans: Integrative health programs recognize that every person is unique, so treatment plans are tailored to everyone's specific needs, preferences, and circumstances. This may involve a combination of conventional medicine, complementary therapies, lifestyle changes, and self-care practices.
- Emphasis on prevention: Integrative health programs emphasize preventive measures to promote overall well-being and reduce the risk of illness. This may include education on healthy lifestyle habits, stress management techniques, and strategies for maintaining a balanced mind-body connection.
- Evidence-informed practice: While integrative medicine integrates complementary therapies, it still relies on rigorous scientific evidence and clinical experience to guide decision-making. Treatments and interventions should be supported by research and have a demonstrated safety and efficacy profile.
- Education and empowerment: Integrative health programs strive to educate patients about their health conditions, treatment options, and self-care practices. By empowering individuals to make informed decisions, they aim to enhance individuals' ability to manage their health effectively.
- Continuity of care: Integrative health programs often promote ongoing relationships between health care providers and patients to ensure coordinated and consistent care. This may

involve regular follow-up visits, communication between providers, and access to resources for continued support and education.

It is important to note that the organization and structure of integrative health programs can vary between different health care settings and institutions. These principles provide a general framework, but specific programs may have unique features based on the expertise and resources available to them.

Qualities of Successful Complementary Care Programs and Services

Successful complementary care programs and services often exhibit several key qualities. A successful program embraces an integrative approach, combining complementary therapies with conventional medicine. It recognizes the importance of collaboration between different health care modalities to achieve optimal patient outcomes. Successful programs rely on evidence-based practices and continually evaluate the efficacy of their therapies. This ensures that the treatments provided are supported by scientific research and have demonstrated positive results. Quality programs employ well-trained practitioners who possess appropriate certifications and credentials in their specific fields. They maintain a high standard of professionalism, ensuring the delivery of safe and effective care. A successful program places the patient at the center of its approach. It considers their unique needs, preferences, and goals when designing treatment plans. Patient satisfaction and improved health outcomes are driving factors in these programs. Effective communication and collaboration between health care providers are vital. Successful programs encourage open dialogue and coordination between complementary care practitioners, primary caregivers, and other health care professionals involved in the patient's treatment. Processes need to be put in place to ensure that this collaborative communication is facilitated. Tailored treatment plans are developed based on individual assessments. Successful programs recognize that every patient is unique and requires an approach that suits their specific condition, circumstances, and goals. Complementary care programs that take a holistic approach address not only the symptoms but also the underlying causes of health issues. They consider various aspects of well-being, including physical, mental, emotional, social, and spiritual factors. A successful program emphasizes continuity of care, ensuring a smooth transition between different therapeutic interventions or health care providers, if necessary. This helps maintain consistent progress and avoids fragmented or disjointed treatment experiences. It is important to note that these qualities may vary depending on the specific complementary care program or service. Successful programs continuously evolve to adapt to emerging evidence, patient needs, and changes within the health care landscape.

Exemplars of Integrative Care Programs

It is helpful to analyze exemplars of successful integrative care programs. Here are three examples of integrative programs in the United States, along with information on their location, target audience, directors, and positive effects on public health:

- Cleveland Clinic Center for Functional Medicine. Location: Cleveland, Ohio. Target audience: Patients seeking a personalized approach to chronic disease management. Director: Dr. Patrick Hanaway. Positive effects: The Center for Functional Medicine utilizes an integrative and personalized approach to tackle chronic diseases. By combining conventional medicine with evidence-based complementary therapies, they have achieved positive outcomes in patient health. The program focuses on preventive measures, dietary modifications, mind-body techniques, and lifestyle changes, leading to improved patient outcomes and reduced health care costs (Cleveland Clinic Center for Functional Medicine, 2023).
- Duke Integrative Medicine Center. Location: Durham, North Carolina. Target audience: Individuals seeking comprehensive wellness and preventive care. Director: Dr. Adam Perlman. Positive effects: Duke Integrative Medicine takes a holistic approach, incorporating conventional and complementary therapies for optimal health outcomes. Their programs

emphasize areas such as nutrition, stress reduction, physical activity, and mind-body techniques. By addressing the root causes of health issues and empowering individuals to take an active role in their well-being, Duke Integrative Medicine (2023) has witnessed positive results in chronic disease management, pain relief, stress reduction, and overall quality of life improvement.

- Veteran's Health Administration (VA). The VA has been integrating and providing CIT to clients for many years. In 2011 89% of their medical centers offered at least two CITs, and in 2015 this figure jumped to 93% (Cottreau et al., 2015). The VA has moved from a disease-based medical care system to a system that addresses the whole person, with CIT being offered as a core component. It has been reported that some VA centers that provided CITs were extremely successful while others faced challenges. Research was conducted to investigate the reasons for this. Through their research on this issue, researchers have identified nine key factors that facilitated the implementation of CIT integration (Table 10.1, Taylor et al., 2019).

Table 10.1 Factors Facilitating Complementary and Integrative Therapy Implementation

Having a strategic plan for complementary integrative therapies (CITs) and a CIT steering committee
Offering the individual types of CIT into one program rather than spreading over multiple departments
Including CIT program leads and practitioners who are "strong, professional, enthusiastic, and perseverant" (p. S54)
Obtaining leadership support
Having providers who support CIT
The perceptions of clients' attitudes toward CIT
Showing evidence of the effectiveness of CIT
Being a champion of CIT
Marketing effectively CIT programs

Seven common challenges were also identified in the VA system in offering a CIT program. These include challenges in finding qualified CIT practitioners, insufficient or inconsistent funding, gaining patient access, difficulties in coding and documenting CIT use, having inappropriate space to deliver CITs, insufficient CIT practitioners and support of staff's time, and the health care cultural and geographic environments (Taylor et al., 2019).

In this author's experience of opening a hospital based freestanding CCC in a very conservative community, the cultural and geographic environment was the most challenging element and was somewhat limiting. Much teaching was required to get the public informed on appropriate therapy use. This requires extra resources in terms of a dedication of time and the financial support involved. Further, it was a challenge to get staff in the hospital to become knowledgeable and amenable to allow the integration of CITs in the in-patient setting. Many seminars, meetings with staff members, and leaders in different departments had to be conducted, and at times buy-in was never fully achieved. There are some individuals who are fearful of therapies, which are energy based or spiritual in nature, and this can lead to great resistance. This includes CITs such as therapeutic touch, cranio-sacral therapy, meditation, yoga, and tai chi, to name a few. If these therapies are offered in some geographical areas that are extremely conservative and that lack general knowledge about CITs, it can be more difficult to offer a successful CIT program. The groundwork must be done in educating all members of the community first.

These programs demonstrate the effectiveness of an integrative approach to help meet the holistic needs of their health care consumers. They each have distinct differences but also similar characteristics, which have contributed to their continued growth and success. Planning for CIT roll-out with concrete short-term and long-term goals goes far in guaranteeing the success of a program. Although firm goals are important, one cannot be afraid to make changes as circumstances permit to enhance the CIT offerings that are in place. For example, if an enthusiastic CIT wants to be involved and there is room for another line of CITs, it may be in the CIT program's best interest to allow another offering. Gathering data on what clients are looking for in terms of CIT type and on the current effectiveness of therapies for managing different symptoms and disease states does much to ensure that CITs will continue to be supported and offered. Having champions to push the integration of CITs, organization support, and qualified practitioners are common themes that can be mimicked to guarantee support for any CIT startup. Of course, it never hurts to have substantial financial backing for a CIT integration project, so obtaining data to show need and effectiveness helps in acquiring this sort of support. As more CIT programs are offered, it will open the door to acquiring more information regarding what contributes to a CIT program's success.

Discussion Questions for Your Consideration

1. Can you explain the key components you would consider when critiquing the quality of an integrative care center?
2. How would you evaluate the effectiveness of the integrative care services provided at a center, and what indicators might you look for?
3. In your opinion, what are the most crucial factors to consider when assessing the safety and security of patients receiving care at an integrative care center? Why?
4. Expand on these questions in a 300- to 400-word essay.

Experiential Activities

Visit a local complementary integrative care center and take a tour. Interview the director and ask them the following questions:

1. What led you to select the services that you offer at your center?
2. Have you ever run into any obstacles in providing CITs to the public?
3. What types of challenges do you face in running your center from day to day? Can you give me some examples?
4. What direction do you see your center moving to in the future? For example, will your services change in any way? Is there something new that you would like to add to your center, or would you like to move in a different direction in some way?
5. What are the greatest benefits that your center has for those who come here?

6. Do you have any communications with client's primary care providers regarding the care the client receives here, or do you operate entirely independently?

Reflect after your visit. Were there any safety concerns that you noticed at this center? What did you like most about the center? How was this center structured? Do you have any suggestions for improvement of the center? Draft a short essay, no more than three pages, reporting on your visit.

References

Cleveland Clinic. (2023, October). Center for Functional Medicine. https://my.clevelandclinic.org/departments/functional-medicine

Duke Integrative Medicine Center. (2023, October). Announcements. https://www.dukehealth.org/locations/duke-integrative-medicine-center

Taylor, S. L, Boton, R., Huynh, A., Dvorin, K., Elwy, R., Bokhour, B. G., Whitehead, A., Kligler, B. (2019). What should health care systems consider when implementing complementary and integrative health lessons from Veterans Health Administration? *The Journal of Alternative and Complementary Medicine, 25*(1), 552–560.

Index

D

E

F

G

H

N

O

About the Author

Catherine Stiller began her search on the effect of complementary and integrative therapies when she first served as Director of Complementary Care for Saint Vincent Health System in Erie, Pennsylvania in the late nineties. She is a registered nurse, a therapeutic touch practitioner, and has researched the effect of therapeutic touch on fibromyalgia pain and anxiety, earning her Ph.D. in nursing at the Frances Payne Bolton School of Nursing in Cleveland, Ohio in 2006. Catherine currently serves on the American Holistic Nurses Association Research Committee. She has taught nursing both in person and online for the last 35 years and is a certified nurse educator.

www.ingramcontent.com/pod-product-compliance
Ingram Content Group UK Ltd.
Pitfield, Milton Keynes, MK11 3LW, UK
UKHW021831270726
14058UKWH00001B/87